TAKE IT
to HEART

ALSO BY PAMELA SERURE

*3 Days to Vitality: Cleanse Your Body,
Clear Your Mind, Claim Your Spirit*

TAKE IT
to HEART

The Real Deal on Women
and Heart Disease

PAMELA SERURE

MORGAN ROAD BOOKS

New York

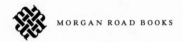

MORGAN ROAD BOOKS

PUBLISHED BY MORGAN ROAD BOOKS

Published in the United States by Morgan Road Books,
an imprint of the Doubleday Broadway Publishing Group,
a division of Random House, Inc., New York.
www.morganroadbooks.com

Morgan Road Books and the M colophon
are trademarks of Random House, Inc.

This book is not intended to take the place of medical advice from a trained medical professional. Readers are advised to consult a physician or other qualified health professional regarding treatment of their medical problems. Neither the publisher nor the author takes any responsibility for any possible consequences from any treatment, action, or application of medicine, herb, or preparation to any person reading or following the information in this book.

BOOK DESIGN BY AMANDA DEWEY

Library of Congress Cataloging-in-Publication Data
Serure, Pamela.
Take it to heart: the real deal on women and heart disease / by
Pamela Serure.
p.   cm.
1. Heart diseases in women—Personal narratives. 2. Heart diseases
in women—Popular works. I. Title.

RC685.C6S455 2006
362.196'120082—dc22
2006041962

ISBN-13: 978-0-7679-2310-1
ISBN-10: 0-7679-2310-3

Printed in the United States of America

10 9 8 7 6 5 4 3 2 1

First Edition

To . . .

The power of my heart, and to all the other women who hold that power inside their hearts

My Parents Gloria and Hy, for all their love and for seeing me through this ride called my life

My true Heart ON, my puppy, my ally, Habebe, who on a daily basis opens my heart

What a heart-on is:

The place where intuition is born, the message that comes from the heart, the place where the heart turns everything else on, the expression of the authentic self, the ultimate "aha!" of the heart and soul.

CONTENTS

Foreword by Alexandra Lansky, M.D.   *xiii*

1. WAKE-UP CALL   *1*

2. OVER MY DEAD BODY   *29*

3. THE FAMILY BUSINESS   *61*

4. THE BOOK IS SEALED   *89*

5. THE THREE STOOGES OF HEALING:
   DISBELIEF, DENIAL, AND DEPRESSION   *119*

6. THE WHITE SALE: EVERYTHING
   MUST GO   *149*

7. WHERE IT STOPS, NOBODY KNOWS   *169*

*Appendix. Straight from the Heart: Resources for Women
with Heart Disease*   *199*

Acknowledgments   *221*

FOREWORD

It was Christmas Eve. Sally was sitting down to dinner with her husband and her two boys, age six and seven. She apologized that she wasn't feeling well. She had been running around all day, getting the house and dinner ready for the holiday. Sally sat in silence for a while, trying to ignore what was going on in her body, but the pain in her stomach and mid-chest area kept getting worse. Her husband noticed that she couldn't catch her breath, and he asked, "Sally, what's wrong?" She said she had no idea. So John put Sally and the children into the car and managed to get them to the emergency room before Sally collapsed.

I was the intern on call that Christmas Eve. When Sally arrived at the ER, she was having a massive heart attack. She was only thirty-six years old, a gorgeous, active tennis player and the mother of two beautiful children. Her family couldn't believe what was happening to her, nor could I. They stood there in stunned silence as I and the other doctors started compressing Sally's chest right there on the pavement of the parking lot, desperate to get her heart beating again. Thankfully, we did. I lost track of Sally after she was transferred to another hospital, but I heard that she went on to receive a heart transplant. I like to believe that she is among us today, enjoying her children, now grown.

Heart disease is devastating, and yet few women are aware of the threat it presents to them. The number of women's lives claimed by heart disease continues to rise each year in the face of a steady decline in the disease witnessed in men. Heart disease remains *the single leading cause of death among women,* and more women than men in the United States die of it. *Heart disease is your greatest health risk. This is a fact. Friends, sisters, mothers, daughters, and wives—this disease will unavoidably affect you, your life, and your family.*

Unfortunately, heart disease is greatly stigmatized for women. As a result, it does not receive the attention it deserves—either from women or from the medical community—and with tragic consequences. Women delay seeking medical treatment, delays that could mean the difference between life and death. Potent preventive and therapeutic alternatives have proven beneficial to women, yet women are frequently excluded from clinical trials, and doctors often fail to apply these practices to women.

Doctors commonly misdiagnose and undertreat women with heart disease even when they present with classic symptoms. One of my patients experienced progressively worse neck and jaw pain whenever she climbed stairs. She had seen a dentist, two dental surgeons, and undergone two molar extractions before coming into my office. These doctors should have noted sooner that the root cause of her pain was actually heart disease and not the need for a root canal. Another patient of mine with heart disease was hospitalized and treated repeatedly for asthma, even though she did not respond to the customary asthma treatment.

The preconceived notion that women are somehow "protected" from cardiovascular disease is simply wrong. A woman older than fifty-five with high cholesterol, high blood pressure, and a family history of heart disease is at risk and should be under active management. The presence of diabetes, regardless of age, is a stronger risk factor for women than for men and warrants very aggressive preventive care. Approximately $200 billion is spent each year on cardiovascular health, with only six cents of every dollar spent on prevention. Spending more on educating, studying, and treating younger women now would be a wise investment in the future.

All of these factors explain why *Take It to Heart* is such an important and timely book. As a female cardiologist, raising awareness about the dangers of heart disease in women, advocating more research and better treatment for women, and reducing the numbers of women who die from this disease are my passions. I feel incredibly fortunate to have crossed paths with Pamela Serure, whose energy and work is inspirational. In this book, she shares not only her most heartfelt experiences with her own heart disease but also the stories of many other women, as well as medical facts and segments written by leading experts in the field. Every woman in America should read *Take It to Heart*. It is the most powerful weapon I've found yet in our battle against heart disease in women.

Ultimately, my goals and Pamela's are one and the same. We are striving to improve women's health and well-being today and for generations to come, so that never again will two young boys have to witness the heart attack and collapse of their mother from this preventable disease.

— ALEXANDRA LANSKY, M.D.
Director of Clinical Services for the Center for Interventional Vascular Therapy at New York–Presbyterian Hospital, Associate Professor of Clinical Medicine at Columbia University Medical Center, and Medical Director of the Women's Health Initiative at the Cardiovascular Research Foundation

1.

WAKE-UP CALL

I always thought of my life as a real heart-on.
That is, up until the day my heart turned off.

—PAMELA SERURE

I am writing about a broken heart. Not the variety that comes from a disrupted family or a disillusioned love affair, nor the kind brought about by a longing that has never been fulfilled. Not that I haven't experienced those; I assure you I have endured all the varieties. But this particular story is about a different sort of heartbreak—the heartbreak caused by heart disease.

The Heart Truth

Heart disease is the number-one killer of American women.

—AMERICAN HEART ASSOCIATION (AHA), 2005

I have always thought of my heart as being *on*—vibrant, open, optimistic, and exuberant. Ever since I was a kid, I had believed that everything was possible. I knew that I was wanted and loved by my parents and my larger family, and that knowledge gave me the confidence to pursue my dreams. Being a born Scheherazade, I enjoyed playing to the crowd and lived for adventure.

I never married or had children, because I didn't want to give up my freedom. Looking back on those choices, I recognize the profound emotional gratification I deprived myself of. Nevertheless, as life progressed, my various careers— designing jewelry, merchandising and creating fashion, and developing innovative health concepts—brought me much recognition and many accolades and awards. I felt satisfied (to a point) and successful (to a degree). Many of my friends became famous and I played on the fringes of celebrity.

In my early forties, I wrote my first book, *3 Days to Vitality,* based on my healthy detox program, Get Juiced. I had become a juice-fasting guru among the Hampton set and was already two decades into meditation and yoga, but my internal mantra was "Do more—be more, have more." I still binged on stress whenever and wherever it appeared. It was the diet of choice for women on the fast track, and I was a born sprinter. Stress was a habit I sipped like a triple latte. But just like caffeine, stress provided only a false sense of being energized, and it barely kept me afloat. Also, it brought along with it its constant companions: cortisol, the stress hormone, which ravages the body, and adrenal fatigue, a burnout condition all of us stress junkies eventually experience. In never stopping, never taking no for an answer, never being or doing enough, I was wearing my heart out while my mind kept on going. But I wasn't paying attention. Sound familiar?

I genuinely liked the person I was. I was at an exhilarating point in my life and I still believed that I could do anything . . . up until the day when my heart turned *off.* That is when I had to surrender the "More" and "Go"—the two commands by which I'd operated my life. Heart disease became my wake-up call: I had to stop listening to that prodding mantra and pay attention to the messages from my heart that I had ignored. Heart disease shocked me into accepting that my relentless drives had been serviced by all the emotions I had kept in check for years: doubt, fear, judgment, and a feeling of not being good enough. Those drives had kept me away from a deeper place of rest and gratitude in my life. And I needed to get to that place. I needed to put on the brakes and get down to the business of healing.

♡ *Heart disease is the body's way of saying stop: Stop driving yourself; stop overreaching; stop trying to fix the world. Just stop whatever it is that you were so hell-bent on doing and breathe.*

All my dreams, confidence, creativity, and healthy living could not protect me from where my heart was about to take me . . . which was not, as I'd often hoped, to the love of my life or to all my dreams fulfilled, but to a 99 percent blockage of my arteries and triple bypass surgery. I had *heart disease,* the old man's disease. The disease for people who don't take care of themselves. The disease of denial for young and vital women. I was no longer feeling the glow of the Golden Child, nor like a lucky person, nor even special. When you feel special, you think nothing can penetrate your aura, but it's only a delusion. As it turned out, I was so much more than *not special;* I was a cookie-cutter case of a woman with heart disease—the family disease, the stress disease. I was one of every two women living silently with our number-one killer. I was one of the eight million American women whose hearts had turned *off.*

The Heart Truth

One out of 2.5 American women will die from heart disease or stroke.

—AHA, 2005

In the seven years since my first heart event, I've arduously come to terms with what happened. For starters, I finally had to admit that I had a broken heart—from promises unkept, from love unmet, from genes unknown. Second, I had to stop. Stop all the movement, the nonsense, and, above all, the drama that fed my heart disease what it needed to grow. I had to focus instead on attending to my heart daily by savoring the little pleasures, reprioritizing, and re-learning how life wanted to be lived. Finally, I had to break my denial and admit that I had a chronic disease. I had to surrender to the truth that heart disease and I were going to be lifelong partners.

These days, heart disease has all my attention, as it should have yours. Not only do 1 in 2.5 American women have it but we also die from it faster because it's harder to detect in us, we take longer to get care because we don't know what the symptoms feel like, and we don't want to admit to having it because we fear it is a fatal disease and imagine that it afflicts only aging men. But in truth, it is a woman's fate as much as a man's. *Heart disease among women shouldn't be a secret, and I am not keeping it anymore.*

Ten years ago, a famous psychic told me that my destiny in this lifetime was to be a teacher of women. Of all the things I'd imagined becoming in my life and had worked to accomplish, being a teacher was never one of them. And yet here I am, called now to share with women the truth about heart disease. My destiny came in an unexpected way, but it's my destiny nonetheless. I'm writing this story now because I have to; I have no choice but to follow my heart. It has become the true story of my life, as it has become the story of so many women's lives.

Heart Song

CATHY A., *Atlanta, Georgia*

I had my first heart attack at thirty-nine. It was just a hairlike tertiary artery, so I basically ignored it. Told myself it was no big deal. Then at forty-two, I had a massive heart attack. I flatlined thirteen times in two and a half hours. No one in Georgia had ever seen anything like it before. All my major arteries went at once.

The night of my massive heart attack was Tuesday, April 12, 1998. I should've been smarter. I should've known better. Not only had I suffered one heart attack already but I was a rehab nurse at the hospital, so I worked with heart attack and stroke patients all the time. But all I did that night when I started having chest pains was call my mom. I didn't do anything else until 1:30 A.M. on Wednesday, when the big pains hit and I started sweating from places I didn't know it was possible to sweat from. That's when I finally went to the hospital.

You know how sometimes you're watching a movie and it fades to black? I was sitting on the gurney, and I did that. Last thing I thought before I flatlined was,

I'm screwed. I knew I was dying. There was no way I could hurt the way I hurt and survive. I was panicking. I was telling the nurses I worked with, people who knew me, "I'm dying! I'm dying! I'm dying!" They kept saying, "Calm down." I said, "I'm dead." Then I was gone, down for the count. It was a horrific situation. Every time I came back, I'd start talking as if I was having normal conversation, but then I'd flatline again. After six or seven times, they usually let you go. But my friend Darlene, who was working on me, said, "She's fighting, so we have to fight, too." I was lucky to be at a hospital where the nurses were my friends. So the doctors kept going.

When I woke up seventeen hours later in the ICU, I thought I was dead. I heard a funny noise and wondered why it was so dark. I thought, What? I didn't make it to heaven? I could feel my consciousness trying to wrap itself around the trauma. But then as the fog began to fade, I started thinking, Wow, I'm alive? I was amazed, as were all the nurses.

I put 99 percent of the blame for my heart disease squarely on my own shoulders. I'd spent many years smoking, starting when I was seventeen. Even when I had that minor heart attack at thirty-nine, I quit for only a year, and then I started smoking again. I was also a heavy pot smoker. I drank a lot. I was overweight. I didn't exercise other than to get up to go to the fridge. I didn't have enough respect for myself to pay attention to the gravity of cardiovascular disease. I knew all about heart disease because I worked with people who had it. Yet still I'd say, "I'll drink and smoke till the day I die." And I was true to my word, because I did die, but I was resurrected. The doctors said, "We don't know why you're here." I said, "You know you're in trouble when you go to heaven thirteen times and they put up a sign that says 'Do not disturb.' You know God's got some greater mission for you to accomplish in life."

Since waking up from my heart surgery that day, I've taken my medicine, changed my diet, quit smoking and drinking, and started exercising. I was horrified to know that I had really killed myself.

But I still had battles to fight in this war. After the triple bypass, I did well for about two months, and then I started having trouble again. I'd hurt real bad from angina when I lay down at night, and it would wake me up in the morning. I told my doctors, "Something is wrong." But you know, I'm afraid that when male doctors in particular see a woman coming in time and again for the same problems, they say, "Oh, you're just having anxiety. You're making it up." I kept saying, "Bull. You really need to listen to me."

Let me tell you something that I find incredible, so that women who read this will never, ever let their doctors dismiss them again. On the Friday night before my third heart attack, I told the doctor that I wasn't feeling well. He kept me overnight on an IV drip. On June 11, the following day, another doctor came in and said, "I really haven't read your case file, because it's too thick and I don't have time, but I don't see anything indicating that you're having heart problems." I'd thrown up, which is a classic symptom for women. I had a headache. But he said, "I don't see anything. I really think we've got a case of hypochondria here. I'm sending you home." I said, "Something is wrong." He said, "I don't see anything that indicates that." When the nurse came in to disconnect me from the IV, she said, "The doctor wrote an order for you to go home. If you don't leave, your insurance won't pay for it." So I left. I was furious. I said, "I'll be back."

The very next day, June 12, I told my husband to take me to the hospital. I was really hurting. I couldn't manage with the sublingual nitroglycerin. As soon as the doctor ran the EKG, he was barking orders like an army sergeant. The doctor from the day before walked in and started screaming about how I was a hypochondriac and got sent home. But the ER doc said, "Come look at this." He showed him my EKG. Then they both started calling for a cardiac ambulance to take me to a bigger hospital. When I got there, they said, "Gee, we're sorry, but you've had another heart attack." All that first doctor had to do was keep me in the hospital for another twenty-four hours of observation, but he'd dismissed me because I was a woman. He thought I was being stupid or over-reacting, so he sent me home.

My husband and I were furious. My body was going to do what it did, and I take responsibility for my heart disease. But when that doctor dismissed me, I was off-the-charts angry. Arrogant doctors think they know more about us than we do! When I got back to that hospital, I said to the doctor who'd told me I was a hypochondriac, "You're fired."

Luckily, God still wanted me around. I survived my third heart attack and more. In December of 1998, one of the arteries they bypassed closed, and I was on the edge of a fourth heart attack. The doctors put a stent in, then another. They said, "You're going to continue to have cardiac episodes like this until your heart stops. We don't believe you'll live another year." They sent me to a psychiatrist to help me deal with dying. I said, "Are you God? I don't need help dying! I've already done that a couple of times. I need help living." I told him to leave. God didn't put me through all this in order to die; I knew that much.

In March 1999, I started chelation. I'd been con-suming one hundred milligrams of nitroglycerin sub-lingually per week and I couldn't walk to the bathroom without hurting. But after a year of chelation and a regimen of omega-3 fatty acids, vitamin E, and coenzyme Q10, I wasn't even taking nitroglycerin. I was cleaning my house, vacuuming, sweeping, and taking showers without fear of keeling over. I even got a part-time job. I'm fifty years old now and I plan on sticking around for a long time to come.

I have to take responsibility for the fact that I have these heart problems because of my own behavior. But I have two children, lots of friends, and lots of things I want to do. And I don't want to go yet. So I had to find a way to love myself, to fight to stay here. That meant accepting certain things: No, you don't drink, you don't get high, and you don't smoke, because you like breathing a whole lot more. I had to empower myself to live. This is my choice, my destiny. *Choice* is the word. It's your choice. Some people tell me that sounds hard. Well, how much harder is it to leave your kids behind?

The thing for me is that now I don't have bad days, ever. I had a bad day once. It killed me. When I woke up, I understood what God was telling me about a good day. You've got this moment only. Every morning when I wake up and I'm still on this earth, it is a good day. It is an absolutely great day. Anything that happens in between, that's just a thing. I don't holler; I don't scream. I used to get all upset, because I have that type AAA personality. Now when someone honks a horn, I say, "Love you, too. Peace." I don't worry about any of the small stuff. I invest in myself, and if I do that, then I'm investing in everyone I love and adore. You have to entitle yourself, give yourself permission to live a good life.

I go around to schools now and give talks to kids about my experience. I tell them, "Here's what I learned. The dope dealer wasn't at the hospital, the guy at the liquor store wasn't at the hospital, and Phillip Morris didn't send a rep to say hi. You're just money to them. It's an interesting thing. I can laugh at it now." They say, "How can you?" I say, "Why not laugh? I'm not mad at them, and I'm not mad at me. I just wanted to learn and to live. And I did."

Not only did my bypass surgery open the passages to my heart; it opened my eyes. For it was then I learned that heart disease is the silent enemy in our midst, killing more American women than all the forms of cancer combined. And yet I also discovered that most women have no idea that heart disease is our number-one killer. Nor that the symptoms of heart problems in women often differ completely from the chest-clutching Hollywood version of a heart attack that manifests itself in men. Nor that many women today are struggling to recover from their heart events—their heart-offs—by putting on a brave face in spite of their depression, turmoil, and shame. As women, we're amazing, strong, and nurturing. How else to ensure our legacy but to become proactive and take on heart disease as our biggest enemy?

The Heart Truth

Only 13 percent of American women view heart disease as a health threat.

—AHA, 2005

Unfortunately, women aren't the only ones unaware of the dangers of heart disease. Many medical professionals discount the disease in women because it has been taken hostage by men. Men, whose symptoms are clear and who get checked regularly for heart problems. Men, who benefit from having had many medical studies conducted on them alone. Men, for whom heart-attack rates have declined in the past few years, while they've risen in women! As a result, women are going into hospitals, complaining of shortness of breath, a burning sensation in their chest, back, or neck, and jaw pain, and they're being told they're suffering from anxiety and are sent home—sometimes *even during a heart attack.* We are receiving improper treatment and inaccurate diagnoses day after day, time after time, woman after woman, and we're dying because of it. It's shocking but true.

Heart Song

FELICE L., *Las Vegas, Nevada*

I was diagnosed with a heart murmur when I was seven years old. That's what they called it back then, anyway. The cardiologist wasn't too concerned. He told my mom to have my heart checked once a year, and so she did. I had to take antibiotics every time I went to the dentist, but it was no big deal. When I got pregnant at twenty-two, the cardiologist told me I now had mitral valve prolapse (MVP). I said okay. I made it through the pregnancy just fine.

Over the next couple of decades, I continued to see the same cardiologist. When I was in my thirties, I started going in twice a year because my MVP was getting worse. Then when I was about thirty-eight years old, I was diagnosed with high blood pressure and put on all different kinds of meds.

Then in 2002, I started to see my ankles were swelling up—and I mean swelling. I said to my cardiologist, "My feet are swollen. I'm tired. I don't know what's wrong." He said, "Don't worry about it. Get heavy-duty socks. Put your feet up." I was working in the travel industry. I said, "How am I supposed to put my feet up at work?" So he put me on diuretics. But I kept getting weaker and weaker. I was seeing my doctor every three months now, and things were only getting worse. I called the ER a few times on the weekend because my legs and arms were so swollen. I said, "Dr. T., I'm getting weaker." He said, "It's edema from your high blood pressure. I'm going to put you on some different diuretics."

Now, I've always exercised my whole life, so I was very fit. But I got to the point where I couldn't even get up for work. My family kept telling me to get a second opinion. But I loved Dr. T. He'd been my doctor since I was a kid. He was in his sixties, and he'd give me a big hug every time I went into the office. And yet my whole body was swelling up and he was doing nothing. So in June 2004, I finally went for a second opinion.

Well, was that ever the right decision. I found a fabulous cardiologist. Within a week, he had diagnosed that I suffered from MVP regurgitation, edema throughout my whole body, and coronary heart failure. He said, "I would give your valve maybe six months more. If you don't have surgery, you're going to have a heart attack." So old Dr. T. literally had been killing me. My new surgeon thinks that had I stayed with him, I would've died within a year.

My surgery is coming up soon. They're going to

replace my mitral valve. But right now, I'm barely getting through the days, I'm so tired. I get up, then go right back to sleep. I feel like I'm eighty years old. My doctor says it will be a long recovery. But at least I'll be on the road to recovery.

A lot of women with heart disease think they're just going through menopause. We trust our doctors, but they often dismiss heart issues in women. It baffles me how my doctor repeatedly missed what was going on with me, even though I had a history of heart problems from childhood! Look out for the signs yourself. Be aware that you might have heart disease.

I didn't know any of this until I had open-heart surgery myself. Even then, it took awhile to break my denial. When I realized the truth, I felt compelled to make communicating the facts about heart disease among women my highest priority.

While I am aware that I'm imparting these warnings in a somewhat alarming and high-pitched manner, I must say that a heart event is traumatic and warrants the attention. But as with all traumas, I discovered something rich to learn from this one. First of all, I've found that heart disease offers a tremendous source of bonding for women of all ages, interests, and backgrounds. While this disease is insidious, I believe we can choose to see it as something that can serve to help women everywhere turn their hearts *on*. Second, I've discovered that heart women, being all heart, typically become ferocious advocates once we know we have the disease and begin to recover. We fight for ourselves because we recognize that it is truly our birthright to be happy, healthy, and get the care we need and deserve. Finally, there is a component of heart disease that allows us to take a more intimate look at ourselves. For me, heart disease has served as a pathway to appreciating my inner life and myself more deeply, with a new compassion and sweeter joy. It has set a pace by which I can live truly.

♡ *When we live life according to the heart's dictates,*
 we're both mesmerized by the fluidity of surrender
 and terrified by the loss of control.

The thing is, even if you don't have heart disease now, someone close to you probably does or will soon: your sister, your best friend, your mother, your colleague. It's a fact of our modern lifestyle. Dealing with or preventing heart disease is not just about reducing fat intake or getting more exercise, as many medical books on the topic might suggest. We also need to concern ourselves with gaining real knowledge about all the complicating factors, including family history, the way we metabolize stress hormones, and our responses to disappointment and anger. My heart disease resulted from a combo of factors, layered like the deli sandwiches renowned in New York neighborhoods, a towering compilation of stress and genes. These, it turned out, were and still are the most influential relatives in my life.

We cannot go deaf, dumb, and blind to heart disease just because it's intimidating, frightening, and pervasive. The numbers are growing, but we can shrink them by building awareness of the disease, learning to recognize the symptoms, getting regular checkups, and taking better care of our health by exercising and eating right. The heart is the organ of courage and love. Recognizing its needs should be at the top of our list of priorities. Being heart-savvy is the best facelift in town—not to mention the longest-lasting.

The Heart Truth

Heart disease kills more women than all the forms of cancer combined. Yes, even including breast.

—AHA, 2005

With this book, I seek to galvanize a ministry of women who will, with their wisdom and their own heartfelt stories, help me spread the word about heart disease among their networks of friends and family. I also hope to address many of your questions about heart disease. What is the personality of the disease? What are some of the many and varied symptoms? What's it like to have it? What are the remedies, treatments, and medicines most talked about? How do we live with it? How do we care for it, sleep, eat, and make love when we have it? How do we become closer to its roots in women?

♡ *If it happened to me, then it could happen to you.*

That font of emotion, the deepest, most mystical and magical part of us, the heart is the dwelling place of one's true self. We know we need it to express all that we are, all that we feel, but many times we can't or don't or won't. We keep things secret that fester inside our hearts. Secrets, like plaque, harden and often leave us poised for any enemy to make the body its home. The heart welcomes joy but also carries its opposite, despair. Love claims the biggest piece of our hearts, but sometimes love can go years without expressing itself. Ever wonder why we want to get things "off our chests" when we are in danger of losing someone or ourselves?

Take It to Heart will serve as both recipe and remedy—a cautionary tale for women who are fortunate enough to have healthy hearts, and a source of comfort and support for the more than one-third of American women who are dealing with the disease in their lives right now or who each day are finding out that they have it. This book will not censor facts or feelings, although it's neither a political statement nor a blame game. Rather, this is a story from one woman to another, the only kind that spreads. I share what I've learned on my journey: what I had to change, what new and enduring truths I needed to incorporate into my life. The tool that served me best in my healing, that gave me the stamina I needed to travel this difficult road, was my humor. I hope that you will find this book a personal, open, and honest discussion of all the physical, emotional, and spiritual aspects of living with this disease as a *woman*.

While my personal journey serves as the backbone of *Take It to Heart*, I've asked women of all ages, backgrounds, shapes, and sizes to share the stories they carry, and they have answered soulfully, truthfully, and, most important, willingly. You'll find their Heart Songs peppered throughout the book. I've also asked cutting-edge doctors in the field today to enlighten us as to the different faces and phases of this disease, from symptoms and diagnosis to prevention and recovery. I have included "Heart On" sections to help satiate our hungry hearts, heal our broken hearts, and strengthen our healthy hearts.

The Heart Truth

Eight million American women have heart disease.

—AHA, 2005

In order to prevent, live with, and even embrace the reality of heart disease, we must learn to move to the rhythm of a different heartbeat. We must pick our battles, lest they be our last. We must say what we feel in real time, in case there is no more time later. We must challenge our responses instead of going with typical reactions. We must stop and consider rather than constantly plunging forward and controlling everything. We must allow our minds to rest so that our hearts can be alive. We must appreciate that the little moments often can be the biggest ones. We must discover how to be true to ourselves and love whomever and whatever we love no matter who agrees with us.

♡ *Your purpose is your life, and your life is on purpose when you cheat death.*

As heart women, we have a deeper mission. When we begin our journey, we realize it is indeed a rich expedition into the jungles of our questions and the mountains of our desires, the waters of our tears and the sunshine of our being. I say for myself that my heart chose to turn *off* so that I could really turn it *on*. *Take It to Heart* is my way of living from my heart on out.

Heart Song

JUDY K., *Phoenix, Arizona*

My mother died of a heart attack less than twelve hours after she was sent home from the ER. She shouldn't have died that night. She was the victim of a problem that unfortunately is far too common: doctors ignoring symptoms of heart attacks in women.

My mother was sixty-three when she died, but she looked ten years younger. She was also in incredible shape. A week before, we'd gone walking together and she'd had more energy than I did at twenty-nine.

The day my mom died, she'd been out in the sun. It was a hot day. She started feeling unwell, so she went home to rest. When she still didn't feel better a few hours later, my aunt suggested they visit an urgent-care clinic near the house.

At the clinic, my mother complained to the physician's assistant assigned to treat her, saying she was experiencing tightness in her chest and jaw, pain radiating in her left arm, clamminess, sweatiness, and shortness of breath—all classic signs of a heart attack in a woman. But it was 4:45 on a Sunday afternoon, and I suspect the PA just wanted to get home. He told my mother she was dehydrated from the heat. He prescribed ibuprofen, one of the worst things you can give to someone having a heart attack. (Unlike aspirin, which prevents the clots that cause heart attacks from forming and is considered one of the most important medicines for heart disease, ibuprofen may actually increase the risk of heart attack and block aspirin from working.) Then he told my mother to go home, eat a popsicle to cool off, drink lots of water, and get some rest.

Tragically, my mother took the PA's advice. She went to bed early, complaining that she still felt ill. My grandma, who was in her late eighties at the time, found her daughter dead in her bed the next morning.

I wish my aunt had taken my mother to the hospital instead of to a clinic. I wish my mother had seen a doctor and not just a physician's assistant. I wish the PA had listened to her. I wish that one of the family members with her at the time had known more about women and heart disease. But sadly for us, this was the way things happened, a chain of errors. And my mother, a vibrant, beautiful woman, passed away as a result.

Since then, I've learned a lot about women and heart disease. Every day in the United States, it's like one planeful of women crashes into the ground and dies as a result. Given our family history, my sister and I are now getting our hearts checked regularly.

But the main message I have to share with other women is this: Stand up for yourself and take action. If you think there's even a remote chance that you're having a heart attack, insist on having a full set of tests. Don't worry that your family or the doctors will think you're silly if you're wrong. Take the time to get yourself checked out. If you aren't completely satisfied, ask to speak to a second physician.

You have to take responsibility for your own care. It's worth your time and money if it means that you're going to be alive the next day. My mother was not alive the next day, and I miss her.

HEALING THE HEART

Quiz: Are YOU at Risk for Heart Disease?

By MATTHEW BUDOFF, M.D., cardiologist, associate professor at UCLA Medical Center

PHYSICAL FACTORS
- **Are you overweight?**
- **Do you carry most of your excess weight in the stomach region?**

- Do you eat processed and/or fast food more than twice a week? Have you been doing so for years, or perhaps your entire life?
- Are potatoes, carrots, and other starchy or sugary vegetables your primary sources of vegetable matter?
- Do you have high blood pressure?
- Do you have high cholesterol levels?
- Do you sweat heavily during or after the slightest physical exertion?
- Do you often have gastric trouble, acid reflux, or heartburn?
- Are you diabetic?
- Do you smoke? Have you ever smoked for more than a year?
- Do you have a family history of heart disease?
- Are you in menopause, postmenopause, or perimenopause?
- Do you take hormones?
- Do you ever experience pain in the jaw, neck, or shoulder region that is unexplained?
- Are you an emotional eater who prefers fatty foods?

EMOTIONAL FACTORS
- Have you been hiding something in your life for a long time?

- Have you had more than four unsuccessful love affairs/relationships?
- Do you have blue moods more than three times a week?
- Does something feel incomplete inside you no matter what you do?
- Do you dislike your body in whole or in parts?
- Do you admonish yourself for most of your actions?
- Do you often feel anxious, angry, or sad—or all three?
- Have you been depressed for more than three years?
- Is loneliness a factor in your life?
- Have you been heartbroken more than twice?
- Do you have fits of unexplained anger or rage?
- Do you feel as though your life hasn't turned out the way you wanted and expected it to?

MENTAL FACTORS
- Do you feel as though you're never satisfied?
- Do you drive your body too hard?
- Do you need to be in control?
- Do you fly off the handle easily?
- Do you overthink each situation?
- Is everything you do wrought with stress?
- Do you feel as though there's never enough time?
- Do you have an "off" button inside yourself that you can't seem to find?

- Do you worry endlessly about everything?
- Do you have a sense of futility about the future?

If you answered yes to three or more of these questions, it's time to get into a conversation about what's going on with your heart. Please visit your doctor for a heart exam.

2.

OVER MY
DEAD BODY

The body we have, with its aches and pleasures,
is what we need to be fully human, awake, and alive.

—PEMA CHODRON

How do I really pop this book open, the book about one of the most significant passages of my life? Should I simply allow the words to flow out and breathe on their own, like the vapors from a just-corked bottle of peppery Syrah? Should I pry them out like sardines folded tightly into one another in their briny placenta? Or should I be witty to help assuage the feelings inside?

I think I will begin simply by telling you that I am a woman—the same as you in many ways, but of course not exactly the same. As women, we know that we already have shorthand with one another, so I will start from there. We know what life feels like inside our bodies, how it all works when it works and how it feels when it doesn't. We know that sensation in our throats right before we want to scream, and that slow burn in our eyes when we're holding back our tears. We know how to sneak forbidden treats like lifelong thieves, and how to fain perfect innocence upon their disappearance. We know every inch of our naked bodies and still see the flaws above the perfections. We know verses of excuses and chapters on forgiveness. We just know.

♡ *For women with heart issues, honesty really comes to the forefront. It's as if clearing the plaque out of your arteries also rids you of the lies inside. There is a fear, with heart issues looming, that any day might be your last. What if you didn't tell the truth? Whom would you betray in the end?*

Women are a code as much as we are a gender. So it really doesn't matter if I tell you that my hair is short or long, dark or light, if my eyes are blue or green or brown. It shouldn't matter if I tell you that I lost five pounds on the Atkins diet, or that I like dark chocolate more than milk chocolate. I would still be the same as you are or were or will be, sometime or somewhere in your life.

If we were all in a room together, we would probably first check one another out in a superficial way, making passing judgments about one another's clothes, hair, makeup, body firmness, plastic surgery—the full checklist. But then, as time wore on, we would progress to revealing the deeper wounds from our mothers, our lovers, and all the small tragedies we hold so deep within us—the wounds of our hearts, the scars of our souls. No matter the differences, we would bond, sipping wine, laughing, and probably eating a delicious feast someone had prepared. Because when women gather together, we know how to nourish one another with our wisdom, compassion, and humor. We would end our time with a dessert or two to remind us that tomorrow always holds a sweeter promise.

If we sat long enough in that room together, we would certainly notice that we are, as women, more the same than we are different, including the fact that most of us either have heart disease, will have it, or know someone dear to us who has it. I am just one of those voices in a song of many.

The Heart Truth

Heart disease kills 500,000 women each year. That's more than one every minute.

—AHA, 2005

Heart Song

JOAN B., *Honolulu, Hawaii*

I'm seventy years old, but until a year ago I was a powerhouse. I worked full-time and served on several boards. I exercised regularly—I was no marathon runner, but I fit in a mile walk most mornings. I raised four children. My cholesterol count was okay. I wasn't particularly overweight. I wasn't a smoker. But I was menopausal. I'd had a hysterectomy at age sixty-five. Still, I wasn't getting any pains in my chest or arms, anything like you read about as symptoms of heart problems. I just got tired. But hey, I was busy. I was always tired.

Over a period of a month, I started getting a sore jaw at night when I went to sleep. I thought I'd heard about people who would start to grit their teeth as they got older, and so I figured that was happening to me. Anyway, the logical thing to do when you have pain in your jaw is to go to the dentist, right?

My dentist said I could be gritting my teeth at night and not knowing it. So he made a bite plate for me to wear. But even though I wore it every night, the pain persisted. I was taking Tylenol like crazy, and at night I would alternate putting a hot or cold compress on my jaw because the pain was so severe. But it barely helped. It got to be so bad that I dreaded going to sleep.

So I went back to the dentist and told him the bite plate wasn't helping. And he said, "You know what? I'd recommend you go to a cardiologist." I said, "What? You've got to be kidding. Why would I see a cardiologist for my jaw pain?" He said, "Well, many times people go from the dentist's chair to have heart work done. Jaw pain is actually a common symptom of heart problems."

At first, I couldn't believe it, because basically I felt so healthy. But then I started thinking about how both of my parents had died of heart disease in their early sixties. So I went to my internist. I took a stress test and didn't do very well, so he sent me to a cardiologist. To show you how I was handling all this, listen to this: I called the cardiologist and changed my appointment to another day because I had a very important meeting that afternoon. When I finally went in, he said my heart trouble was so severe that he wanted me to come back the next day for an angiogram.

Well, I went straight from the angiogram to quadruple bypass surgery and didn't leave the hospital until ten days later. It turned out that four of my arteries were blocked. But I'm fine now, thank heavens. I feel great, like I have a new lease on life. I went right back to work and I keep myself busy. I am more aware of eating right and exercising now.

I think that women's capacity for pain is great, unlike men's. Perhaps it's because of childbirth. I'd felt like sure, my jaw was sore, but I could take it. I never, ever would have guessed that the pain was associated with heart problems. I had no idea whatsoever that something was going on with my heart. So if not for the smart young dentist, I never would have gone to see the cardiologist, and I would've died of a massive heart attack, just like my father.

I always believed that I would be the first to know intuitively if something were *really* wrong with me. After all, I often say that the greatest tool a woman possesses is her intuition. But now I make an addendum to that proclamation: Intuition works only if you want it to work. Not knowing is sometimes easier than knowing. But the more I muffled my voices, the louder they became. What you resist really does persist.

The Heart Truth

Sixty-four percent of women who died suddenly of cardiovascular disease had no previous symptoms or awareness that they even had the disease.

—AHA, 2005

In my forty-sixth year, I made an impromptu move from Manhattan and the Hamptons for a self-mandated time-off period. Something inside me knew I just needed to go where I had never been before, a place where I could be new to myself and a place that offered me some rest. L.A. seemed to fit the bill.

I wasn't sure if something was wrong with me, but I knew that I was not quite right. It was more than malaise and not quite an illness (I was accustomed to the latter after a lifetime of getting and conquering obscure maladies such as shingles and scarlet fever). And yet after six months in L.A., I still didn't feel well. How could I be "not right" after having moved so far away from home, into the sunshine in my precious Malibu house? How could I be "not right" in a place where every morning I could overlook the idyllic dolphin-strewn playground called the Pacific? How could I be "not right" with the farmer's markets beckoning, feeding my addictions to fresh produce, flowers, and breads? How could I be "not right" when time was all I had now? How was that possible?

♡ *Denial is the internal prosecutor for emotions not ready to be revealed. Denial can make one believe that which is unbelievable.*

My nagging symptoms felt like walking pneumonia (something I'd had many times before), except for the fact that there was this persistent burning in my chest, like heartburn without the garlic, and a pain in my neck, and exhaustion that didn't dissipate no matter how much I rested. I knew this could be due in part to my dwindling visits from the goddess Estrogen, infamous for her spontaneous mood swings, tumultuous hot flashes, and fierce heartbeats. My feeling was that if all the women in the world could synchronize their hot flashes, we would truly give new meaning to the term *global warming*. But at forty-seven, wasn't I a bit young for this harsh a version of the passage?

The Heart Truth

Doctors and patients both tend to misattribute chest pains in women to other causes, such as stress, anxiety, or gastrointestinal problems.

—AHA, 2005

I think it's safe to say that most women always have some symptoms that warrant a checkup. But stress and exhaustion simply have become the modern way of life for us, like having to lose those five extra pounds no matter what the scale says. We're warriors, never thinking about a way or time when we won't feel too tired, too stressed, too put upon. So instead of setting an appointment, we self-diagnose and self-medicate, relying on time-tested remedies like chocolate, facials, white peonies, and shoe shopping. If that doesn't work, we finally, reluctantly, resort to the doctor's visit.

Heart Song

—————

MARILYN K., *Alameda, California*

As best as my current cardiologist can figure it, I had undiagnosed rheumatic fever as a very small child! When I was two, I was diagnosed with a heart murmur. It scared my parents crazy, but since it didn't impinge on any of my activities, all they could do was watch and wait.

At age nine, I started having chest pains, so they took me to a pediatric cardiologist, whose diagnosis was mitral valve regurgitation. My growth spurt was taxing my muscles and my heart, causing "growing pains." However, the doctor decided that I didn't need any meds or surgical repair. So I basically forgot that I had a valve problem and went on to lead a busy life.

Then during my thirties, I started slowing down. I'd have trouble breathing if I ran up a flight of stairs. I had bouts of bronchitis and a hacking cough (even though I'd never smoked). Sometimes I even had heart palpitations. But I attributed these symptoms to high stress and lack of exercise. Anyway, I was too busy at work to deal with doctors, and I felt okay generally. So I continued to push my way through, ignoring how I felt. When I turned forty-four, it finally dawned on me that something was really wrong, and at long last, many months, if not years, after I should have, I scheduled a heart exam.

I went on my lunch hour to have the EKG. It was supposed to be a baseline check. I knew I had a heart murmur, but my doctor wasn't worried. "We'll just check this out as a precaution," he said, "and then I'll refer you to an allergist to see what's causing your wheezing."

The technician was real chatty as he examined the left side of my heart, but he completely stopped talking when he switched sides. He became so upset by what he saw that he literally ran out of the room to get the cardiologist. Meanwhile, I was starting to get annoyed at how long things were taking.

Soon the cardiologist, a nerdy-looking young fellow, came in, looked at the tape, listened to my heart, and broke the news without an ounce of sensitivity. "You've got a leaky valve and it needs replacement. You'll have to have open-heart surgery very soon." I nearly laughed out loud! I had visions of "cracking open the hood," like when your car overheats and you have to pull over by the side of the freeway. I was so surprised that I practically shouted, "You're kidding!" In all seriousness, he replied, "I wouldn't kid about a thing like that." Much later, he apologized, admitting to me that he was so thrown by seeing a walk-in patient in as bad shape as I was that he just said the first thing that came into his head.

When I returned to my office after the exam, I checked in with my boss. She asked me how the test had gone and I said, "Not very well, actually. I have a leaky heart valve and it needs to be replaced. I'll have to have open-heart surgery." She blurted, "You're kidding!" and I broke out into hysterical laughter. "That's what I said," I told her.

Long story short: My open-heart surgery was successful and I got a bionic-valve replacement. I have to take Coumadin (a blood thinner) for the rest of my life, and it's been a bit of a roller-coaster ride getting the balance of meds just right. But I recently celebrated the four-year anniversary of my surgery, and I feel great! I feel so grateful to the many people who helped me along the way. I'm so happy to be alive.

What was my body trying to tell me, anyway? Most likely, it was a call to slow down after having just completed a worldwide book tour and a move from the East Coast to the West. You think? But to me, admitting that I was exhausted at this point in my life was not an option. I never knew what would follow that act. It felt far too vulnerable. It felt like I was failing at being me, the only job I'd ever taken seriously. And after years of defending my life and the way I chose to live it, that would have been the white flag of surrender. It wasn't time yet for that, or so I thought. In truth, the white flag had already raised itself; I had no choice in the matter. I was too tired to keep denying it.

The Heart Truth

Just as we all have different ways of laughing and crying, so, too, are our symptoms—the ways in which illnesses make themselves known to us in our bodies— different. But one thing is certain: When the arteries carrying blood in and out of the heart are blocked for a while, you will feel tired. Very tired. *Life*-tired.

Women are used to living in this exhausted state, so it's even more urgent that we become hyperalert to the particular signs of heart disease. We need to know the difference between a bad hair day, or PMS, or a fight with our significant other, or five extra holiday pounds, and the beginning of a disease that now is being tracked in women as young as thirty.

When illness is present, our appetites—for food, sex, fun, energy—all seem to diminish. Depression, stomach and gastric disturbances, restlessness, anxiety, pains in the back, jaw, or neck, and a burning in the chest are some of the key signs of heart disease in women. Women also frequently experience a sense of hopelessness that starts to pervade the spirit. Depression seems like a familiar friend that just moves in to stay for a while and then stays for good. Please pay attention to these signs. Don't just write them off as the everyday side effects of stress. They could be your *wake-up call*. They could save your life.

—DR. JESSE HANLEY

So in time, I caved in. I couldn't ignore this "not right" feeling any longer; I had to see a doctor. At least I found a great one. Dr. Jesse Hanley is a renowned specialist on menopause—which was perfect for my condition. She came out to greet me wearing cowboy boots and a pink-and-turquoise skirt, almost a mini. Wow, L.A. never disappoints! As I barreled through my list of ailments, Dr. Hanley was totally absorbed. It was as if I were a storyteller and she were waiting for a particular ending. The visit was magical. She was real, she listened, and she spoke in a language designed for women's ears—soft, direct, smart, and caring. She was a women's doctor for sure.

Dr. Hanley instantly picked up that I was an energy junkie feeding my habit daily with stress cocktails. She officially welcomed me to the Adrenal Burnout Club, which is what people who run on stress for too long inevitably join at some point in their lives. Forget type A; she said I had the perfect AAA personality required for membership. She introduced me to the idea of naps, saying they would change my life. I smiled at the novelty and simplicity of the idea. New Yorkers don't take naps; we have another latte. She also told me I was in perimenopause and gave me a complete list of remedies, herbs, vitamins, and protocols to deal with that.

But then she did something I hadn't anticipated. She insisted that I have my heart checked. When I questioned her recommendation, she said it was just a feeling she had about me, since my father had some valve and blood pressure issues. "Let's check your heart." I'd never heard that before. But I wasn't concerned. Doctors like to check things out; it's part of the ritual. I told her I'd do the test in a few weeks, after I got back from a trip home to NYC.

The Heart Truth

Certain diagnostic tests and procedures for heart disease are not as accurate in women as in men, so some physicians may avoid using them. These doctors may not detect heart disease in women until later, resulting in an increased risk of heart attack or stroke—and with more serious consequences.

—AHA, 2005

There is never a good time to hear about your impending death, especially when you feel it is untimely. The human being would rather imagine, fantasize, or create the scene than succumb to it. Yet hardly ever is it the way we envisioned. On a daily basis, just like birth announcements, news of death is delivered in the oddest ways. Mine was announced on an ordinary sunny Southern California day at the end of September 1998.

♡ *Illness is a fantastic lens. It offers perspective and foresight at the same time—the ultimate snapshot of a life.*

Shortly after returning to Los Angeles from New York City, I'd taken the CT heart test that Dr. Hanley had ordered, because I now was adding chest pains to my list of ailments. After the test when I got home, I planted myself in the womb of my bedroom. I was gazing inward, thinking about this enormous move I'd made from New York to L.A., from cold to hot, from crazy to calm, from me to not me. I was thinking about my cocker spaniel, Sage, and how she wouldn't let me walk up the hills of Malibu with her. Day after day, she would tug on the leash, till I would eventually give up and go home. Sage was a sage indeed. I was just sitting there when providence entered along with the fresh sea breezes.

The phone rang. On the third ring, I picked up. "Ms. Serure?" the voice asked. The tone instantly set off alarms.

"Yes?"

"The results of your CT scan are terrible," said the voice on the other end of the line. "In fact, they're life-threatening. I've never seen a score this high on a woman your age with your profile. Your arteries are completely blocked and you are at risk of a major heart attack at any moment."

I collapsed inside myself and went deaf to the rest of the conversation. My unlived life circled me as ferociously as the tornado in *The Wizard of Oz*. A heart attack! I had never re-motely considered the possibility of a heart attack. I mean, I'd thought of cancer of course, pneumonia always, even an exotic island disease, but never once, not even in a drama-queen moment or a passionate writing frenzy, had a heart at-tack occurred to me. Here I was with time off in paradise, and hell was my gatekeeper. There was no way that I knew of to process this kind of information, and so my only release was to burst out crying.

Within the next hour, Dr. Hanley showed up at my house, visibly shaken. Given the CT scan results, she con-vinced me to see a cardiologist who was part of the network she belonged to in L.A. *As soon as possible.*

♡ *You always know when something big is knocking.*
whether you choose to answer the door or not, it will
find its way in if it belongs to you.

Two days later, I sat impatiently in a burgundy tufted leather sofa in the cardiologist's office. I stared with glazed-over eyes at the dark green walls checkered with lackluster oil paintings of mallards and cocker spaniels. A Ralph Lauren decor it was not.

What was I doing there, really? I thought of the thousands of remedies I'd swallowed over the years, my commitment to exercise, and my strict organic diet. I recalled the hundreds of hours spent in ashrams, doing yoga, chanting and meditating to ensure my sanity in stressful situations exactly like these. And yet there I was, at only forty-seven. Could I really have heart disease? I wondered.

The Heart Truth

Nearly 13 percent of American women aged forty-five or over have had a heart attack.

—WOMENHEART, 2005

Finally, I was called into the doctor's office, and a-testing we went: echocardiogram, fine; EKG, fine; heartbeat, fine. All systems normal. . . . So what gives? I thought I *knew* I was right. I always like to be right, but in this case, it was especially true. I didn't have heart disease. It was clear to me that something else was going on—something no one had ever seen before. The doctor gave me his standard apologetic speech—better to be safe than sorry, blah, blah, blah. I excused myself to go to the ladies' room and let out a huge sigh of relief.

But like a cue coming from backstage, that persistent burning in my chest reappeared. It wasn't until that precise moment that I actually felt appreciative of being in a doctor's office. He could uncover the source of my symptoms right then and there. Instant gratification—how appealing to a true New Yorker.

I marched back into the doctor's office and said, *"Now. Test me now. I have that burning sensation I was telling you about."* For the first time during the visit, the doctor stirred, moving out of his doctor zone. He repeated what I'd just said about "this burning sensation" back to me three times, in three different ways.

"You have it now?" he asked.

"Yes, test me now while I have it!"

"You have it just walking to the ladies' room and back?" he asked again, a bit more emphatically this time.

"Yes!" I replied. Why was this so difficult for him to understand?

"Just walking across the hall?" (No, I'd joined Cirque du Soleil in the interim.)

"Yes, yes, and yes!" I replied.

"Ms. Serure," he said, looking as serious as an actor playing the doctor part on TV, "I'm afraid we can't let you leave this office."

"What?"

"This burning sensation means that you have unstable

angina and you could have a heart attack just from walking across the room. So I can't let you leave my office."

"What?" I repeated, panic creeping into my voice.

"We must admit you to the hospital immediately," said the doctor. "You could die at any moment."

Hospitalization? Die? Now? "I can't do this!" I shouted. "I have to go home. I have to walk Sage. I have to get my toothbrush. I need my cashmere blankie."

"I'm sorry, that's not going to happen," he said as he placed a wheelchair before me. "We need to get you in *right now.*"

"I swear I'll come back later," I pleaded (meaning later, like after getting three other opinions later, though I did not say that out loud). But apparently my acting and negotiating skills, like my energy levels, were waning, because I was having zero effect.

Within the next five minutes, I was ushered at the speed of the opening minutes of an *ER* episode into St. John's Hospital, a destination a long way from home. On the ride in, faces melted into walls, morphing like computer images, and the sounds and smells became psychedelic. If you've ever had the experience where it takes forever to get admitted to a hospital, watch what happens when the staff members hear the words *heart attack* and see a thin, healthy-looking woman in her forties being wheeled in. Within the time it takes to order a Big Mac and fries, I was hooked up to monitors recording all my bodily functions, bedpan included.

♡ *There ain't no cloud so thick that the sun ain't shinin'*
on t'other side.
                    —*Rattlesnake, an 1870s mountain man*

The Heart Truth

**More women than men die of heart disease each year,
yet women get only 33 percent of the total
angioplasties, stent procedures, and bypass surgeries,
28 percent of the implantable defibrillators, and 35
percent of the open-heart surgeries.**
                    —WOMENHEART, 2005

Hours later, I was in an operating room, being prepped
for an angiogram. A multitude of doctors began their proces-
sion into the room, muttering while taking their positions.
The thumping of my overstimulated heart grew louder and
louder. The characters were all suited up and moving around
like background dancers in a Michael Jackson video. They
gave me five milligrams of Valium, which in my heyday
would have been considered a chai tea, and then they began.
They cut a small pinhole in my groin and snaked a wire with
a tiny camera lens through me to capture the images of
my heart. Kinky! Next, they shot me full of hot liquid chemicals. "The better to see you, my dear" A warming sensation

spread underneath my skin, like taking a nuclear pee. These chemicals provided the doctors with the knowledge they needed, in the colors that mattered, to find out what was *really* going on.

Suddenly, there we were—the doctors, the nurses, and I as a collective—staring at my tie-dyed heart, my sweet broken heart, my exhausted, overworked heart, holding on for dear life. When I saw that image on the screen above me, it was apparent to me that this was all true: My heart had me held captive.

Abruptly, a big man leaned over and whispered in my ear. "Ms. Serure," he said in a hushed tone, as if it were a seduction, "Ms. Serure, I'm John Robertson, chief of Cardiac Surgery here at St. John's. We're all marveling at your condition." Thank God, I thought, an intervention in all this drama, someone finally bearing good news. "I have some bad news that requires all your attention."

Wasn't the news bad enough already? Was I being punk'd?

Finally, this anonymous doctor was seeing me as I had always seen myself: an urban mystic in the flesh. Never give up on being discovered; you just never know when it'll happen! My inner drama queen felt crowned, and nothing could ever compete with the coronation. Nevertheless, this was not exactly how I'd pictured my coming-out party.

"I am going to give you two days to get your family here and your affairs in order. We don't know if you have even two days to live, but I know you will need that time to process this information. You need a triple bypass, which is open-heart surgery to replace three of your arteries. Your main artery is ninety-nine percent clogged and two other arteries are seventy-five percent clogged. We don't understand how you've been managing even to walk around, much less fly on a plane, without having a heart attack so far. You must have some great relationship with God, because frankly, there is really no explanation as to why you're not dead yet."

Two days to sum up a life, a legacy, a destiny? My affairs could take a year or more to put in order. At least the doctors and I agreed on one thing: I was nowhere near the typical profile of a heart patient. This was to be my ultimate betrayal—the betrayal of being all things healthy; the betrayal of thinking "healthy living" supersedes stress and genetic predisposition. And believe me, betrayal by your own belief system and your own body is much worse than any a lover could ever deliver. This had to be wrong. Whose karma had gotten mixed up with mine?

But no matter how hard I tried to deny it, on that redundant sunny California day I finally had to concede that the battle had turned into a war, whether I liked it or not. Heart disease had invaded my body, unfriendly and uninvited. What choice did I have but to enter the ring with my dukes up, ready for the fight of my life? Round one was about to begin.

HEALING THE HEART

Signs and Symptoms of Heart Disease in Women

By JESSE HANLEY, M.D., author of *Tired of Being Tired,*
coauthor of *What Your Doctor May Not Tell You
About Premenopause*

When Pamela Serure first came to see me, she had diagnosed herself—a New Yorker trait, no doubt. She wanted me to confirm her premature entry into menopause. But her symptoms and her diagnosis did not match—not even close.

It was not in my medical literacy to expect heart disease in such a young, vibrant, nonsmoking, thin, healthy woman still having a normal menses, so I did not set out looking for that. But over the course of our appointment, I noticed a few clues as to what was really going on.

As I carefully took down Pamela's medical history, she revealed several important facts: a family history of heart and vascular disease, and a diet heavy in carbohydrates. Even though the carbs Pamela ate were supposedly the best kind (fresh raw fruit juices), the fact is that she had been living on sugar and adrenal (stress) hormones for years—a dangerous cocktail for the heart, according to modern medicine.

Nor did Pamela's labs and menstrual history reveal

menopause. In fact, her symptoms of fatigue and neck pain were suspiciously similar to those for heart disease. Unfortunately, there are no clear-cut symptoms of heart disease in women in general. The classic one—shortness of breath, especially with exertion—can be insidious. Many women and doctors overlook it. Many women even ignore chest pain and simply slow down, as Pamela had been doing.

So I sent Pamela to have an ultrafast CT scan to test for heart disease, although this was before the test was fashionable. Thank heavens I did. It was more sensitive than the subsequent treadmill test the cardiologist gave her, and we may never have recognized the severity of her case without it. I still see the ultrafast CT scan as the best screening test, far more accurate than the standard EKG. Best of all, it is noninvasive. Fortunately, it is rapidly gaining recognition and acceptance.

When the results came back, Pamela's diagnosis of advanced atherosclerosis surprised me as much as it surprised her and all who know her. Good thing my intuition was working that day and that I was paying attention, because Pamela's case served as an excellent lesson for me. Women, after all, are at least as vulnerable as men to heart disease, and given how masked their symptoms can be—as Pamela's were—doctors must review their cases with a heightened sense of importance.

Even though heart disease is the number-one killer of

women, the truth is yet to be revealed to us in a way that engages all of our attention. I am a firm believer that we, the medical community, along with heart disease survivors like Pamela, must find new ways to educate and inspire women to be conscious of everything our hearts are saying. Pamela and I are great friends now, and we consider ourselves warriors on the path toward enlightening women as to the risks, symptoms, and cures of heart disease. Please, pay attention to the signs of heart disease and be an advocate for yourself.

CHECK IT OUT

The Top Five Tests for Heart Disease

BY ALEXANDRA LANSKY, M.D.

1. *Thallium stress test:* nuclear imaging test that shows how well blood is flowing to the heart muscle, usually done postexercise on treadmill (hence "stress" test).
2. *Ultrafast CT scan:* particular type of cardiac tomography that provides cross-sectional images of the chest, including the heart and large blood vessels.

3. *Stress echocardiogram:* ultrasound test given during exercise, which visualizes the heart's pumping action and may reveal lack of blood flow not apparent in other tests.

4. *Perfusion MRI:* magnetic resonance imaging, which uses magnets to look inside the body, resulting in 3-D computer-generated pictures of the heart and large vessels.

5. *Angiogram (most invasive):* small catheter inserted into artery up to heart through arm or groin, then patient injected with radiographic substance; tiny X-ray instrument on catheter shows high-contrast images of arteries.

Be informed. Be proactive. Do something good for yourself. If you're at risk for heart disease, or exhibit any symptoms, please ask for these tests.

HEART ON

Meetings with God

I always believed in God. I always believed something or someone was watching over me, guiding me, and doing for me what I could not or would not do for myself. Not everything came my way or went as planned. Whose life does? And yet I still recognized that God was present in all my actions, whether I had full appreciation for the outcomes or not.

I've had many meetings in my life for many different reasons, but the meetings I have had with God were by far the most important. The first occurred when I was about five years old. I'd been suffering from horrible nightmares. They were probably the garden-variety boogeyman type, but at the time they seemed devastating. My parents took me to a rabbi. He told me in all seriousness and with due authority merely to rub my forehead when I had a bad dream and God would make it disappear. Then he prayed over me and sent me on my way. Miraculously, his suggestion worked time and again.

As often happens, the older I got, the more I imagined that I was in charge and the less time I dedicated to my meetings with God. So when my heart event came around, not only did I need a meeting; I needed an emergency makeup session. The night before the operation, it went something like this: "Dear God, how could I be here? Did I not listen to something I was supposed to listen to? I am so confused about what I believe in right now, God, including you! You have given me so much, so many gifts and so many possible roads to travel. I know that I have abused my energies to achieve success. I know that we have not communicated steadily for a while. I have forsaken a place with you in lieu of a place I thought I wanted more. But it is apparent here and now that I stand with you.

"As you know, I might not make it through this journey you have put before me. If you do keep me, please know I wanted to fall madly in love and produce my greatest works. I wanted to be more benevolent to people and care more for myself. I wanted to take time to understand and appreciate my life. But I need more than these two days. Please, God, I really need your guidance, your grace, and your faith in me now. I do not feel my work is done, but you might. Thy will be done."

Even though in my childlike fearful place, I felt like heart disease was punishment, my heart told me it was a soul call. For most of my life, I'd sought out the newsworthy more than the worthwhile. That's the funny thing about being driven: You can lose the direction of your dreams and they can lose you. And in the end, losing one's dreams is really losing oneself. Those initial months following my open-heart surgery brought me right back into my relationship with my spiritual nature. I felt myself pulled closer to God than ever before, magnetized to the vibration of love. I finally understood the true meaning of surrender.

Naked in my fear, in my belief, in God's and my own grace, I found that eloquent and poetic prayers spontaneously flowed from me each day. I felt like the poet Rumi in his time of grief. What emerged from my heart event was a part of me that allowed my intuition to guide and my mind to obey, not the other way around. Life does get a bit twisted when goals seem to be the prize. Almost dying brought me back to the proverbial realization that my *life* was the real prize. Today, my relationship with God is a partnership that cannot be undone and a meeting that can never be canceled.

♡ *Ten thousand steps a day and ten thousand meetings with God will keep your heart open.*

Heart Song

Alice B., *New York, New York*

I'm just twenty-eight years old. So when I say, "I had heart surgery," people say, "No way! Where's your scar?"

I grew up in Hawaii. I was something of a bookworm, but also fit, healthy, and always outdoors doing stuff. I weighed just one hundred pounds. Why would I ever possibly worry about heart disease?

When I was sixteen, I was talking on the phone with one of my friends, and at some point we were laughing. I remember laughing in a certain way, where I inhaled and my heart started racing. I kept talking. I felt light-headed and weird, but I wasn't worried. I thought maybe I was just excited. I didn't say anything about it to anyone; I just went to bed. When I woke up the next morning, I felt fine. I thought it was an anomaly. But then it started happening more often. My heart would just start going as if I'd run five miles. There was no way I could stop it. I'd go to bed, and the next morning it'd be gone. And yet it became more and more disconcerting.

Eventually, I told my mom. One day, she said she could see my shirt moving because my heart was beating so fast, so she took me to the ER. The doctors weren't sure what was going on. They thought maybe it was some kind of arrhythmia. I was nervous. They tried running all these tests and gave me a heart monitor to wear in school, but still they said, "We don't know." And after awhile, it didn't come back anymore, so I kind of forgot about it.

Then sometime during my freshman year at Stanford, the heart pounding started up again. I would just go to sleep whenever it happened. One day, it got really bad, so I went to the ER. Again, the doctors ran a whole bunch of tests. They told me, "You have supraventricular tachycardia." Then one doctor brought in some med students and said, "This is Alice. She's eighteen and she's got tachycardia. What should we do?" And they said, "Give her adenosine." "What's adenosine?" I asked. "It's a drug that'll stop this heart pounding." So they did. I felt a rush of heat run through me, as if someone had constricted my heart in a medieval torture device. It didn't work. So they said, "Up it to twelve ccs." I said, "Oh my God, you're going to do it again." And they did. The pain was horrible, but it worked. They observed me for an hour and let me go.

I went back to the ER about four more times after that for the same thing. The doctors put me on beta-blockers, saying that would help. But they had to keep upping my dosage because the meds weren't working. Finally, they said, "You can have surgery. That'll take care of this problem once and for all."

The idea of surgery totally freaked me out. But I talked to my parents and did a lot of research. I found out that my doctor was one of the first ever to do this surgery back in the seventies, so I thought, he can't mess it up. I also discovered that I had only a 1 percent chance of dying. It was surgery or medication for the rest of my life, so I said, "Let's try to make this work."

Lucky for me, the surgery went really well. The doctors told me to take it easy for a while, but they said that then I should be okay to do anything. And they were right. My heart problems went away. At first, I would be nervous when I laughed, but soon I discovered that I really *could* do anything. Nothing has happened with my heart since. Everything is fine. Every once in awhile, I'll feel like my heart is about to go nuts, but nothing happens. I actually think the whole experience was kind of cool and neat, kind of crazy. These days, I try to stay healthy, get plenty of exercise, eat well, and take care of myself.

The doctors still don't know what caused my heart problem. I may have been born with it, or it may have developed over time. It may have been genetic, or maybe something happened when I hit puberty and my hormones went into overdrive. Who knows?

These days, I do a lot of volunteer work through the Miss America organization. I try to spread the word that heart disease is the number-one killer of women. I tell women, "You never know when it's going to happen to you. The best you can do is to live a healthy life and go to the doctor regularly to get your heart checked. Also, be really aware of your family history." I go to the doctor every year and get a full physical done. It's tough, a tricky disease. You have to watch out for yourself.

3.

THE FAMILY BUSINESS

In women everything is heart, even the head.

—J. P. RICHTER

Things in my life don't slip past me unnoticed. That's the way I am. And yet I was missing the link that had brought me to this place, the hospital, where I was counting down the days to my open-heart surgery. I could not explain my life to anyone anymore. Nothing I'd ever read in magazines, seen on TV, discussed with doctors, or heard from my friends had ever remotely prepared or even hinted to me that what I'd been suffering from could possibly be *heart disease.* In fact, my friends and I comprised a medical dictionary of issues and ailments. We knew every healer and everything that needed to be healed on the planet. We were the wounded generation, and healing was our journey. But never in any workshop, circle, or ceremony had we healed a woman with heart disease. How could that be? In my mind, the dots did not connect.

The doctors concluded that stress and bad genes were the Gemini twins responsible for my condition. *Heart disease is a family disease,* they told me, from the blood pool your genes jump out of to the way your emotions are metabolized. And the more we looked, the more evidence we found that my family is riddled with heart disease. Only I was the biggest casualty of the bunch. Yes, genes are king.

The Heart Truth

If someone in your family has heart disease, make sure your doctors know this and give you the proper tests and attention.
—AHA, 2005

Still, it was difficult at first for me to accept this explanation that I had the family disease. I mean, I knew that everyone on my father's side of the family had died from some sort of heart condition, but they'd seemed so old, while I was so young. Also, they certainly didn't take care of themselves as well or have the same level of self-awareness as I did. My father had had a valve replaced, but his lungs were so ravaged from years of smoking that he was predestined to suffer some consequences. I'd quit smoking when he'd gotten sick, and that had been years ago. And yes, my mother had soaring cholesterol levels, but she kept on ticking and never had a problem with her heart except for years of uneventful angina. In fact, she had more energy than all of us combined.

I honestly believed that my years of healthy alternative living had bought me a reprieve from the gene pool. Plus, doesn't being the black sheep of the family undo some of the genes that bind? But it turned out that my family was in my blood. There was no escaping it.

♡ *No matter who you are, what you have, what you want, or what you do, it all boils down to where you come from in the end.*

Heart Song

GLORIA G., *Honolulu, Hawaii*

At age fifty-four, I'd been swimming over a mile per day for the past six years. But then I got sick in October 2003, so for awhile I wasn't doing any exercise. When I got over my cold, I thought that I should start swimming again, but I just didn't feel like it. I didn't have the energy. And my skin was looking gray. But I thought these were just normal consequences of getting older.

Then on June 30, 2004, my business partner and I were at the airport, waiting to go to Kauai to visit some clients, when I started to feel overwhelmed with exhaustion. My arms felt tired and I broke into a cold sweat. I didn't feel seriously ill, but I did think maybe I shouldn't get on the plane. Now, I am usually not the kind of person who lets feeling a little sick get in the way of work. So when I said I was hesitating about taking the trip, my colleague agreed that I should go home. As I walked across the airport lobby to get a cab, my briefcase felt so heavy that I had to carry it like a baby, cradled in both arms.

On my way home in the cab, I called my husband to tell him what was going on, and I started to cry. I never cry, so I thought that was strange. Back home, I immediately took my blood pressure, because I've had problems with it ever since I was young, but it was normal. I had no headache or vision problems, but I still felt awful. When my husband got home, he said, "I made you a doctor's appointment for four-thirty P.M." I said, "I need to go to the hospital now." So off we went.

As we walked through the door of the ER, I said, "I think I'm having a heart attack." I don't know why, I just had this gut sense, as well as some awareness of heart disease from reading the news. The receptionist sent me into a room, and it was ten minutes before I saw anyone. The nurse took my blood pressure, which was still normal, as were all my vital signs. Next, the doctor came in to examine me. She said, "We're *sure* you're not having a heart attack, but we're going to do an EKG to rule it out."

So out went the doctor and in came the tech. The moment he attached the leads, his eyes popped out of his head. I said, "What's the diagnosis?" He said, "I'm not allowed to diagnose you, but you're having a massive heart attack right now." He started screaming for the doctor, and a bunch of folks came running into the room. Suddenly, the whole ER was in there with me. They asked me who my cardiologist was, and I said I didn't even have one. By the time one arrived, all my vital signs were going crazy. The cardiologist said the reason my blood pressure had been normal was that I'd been in shock.

The doctors pulled someone off the angiogram table and put me there instead. It turned out that of my four main arteries, one was 100 percent blocked, two were 95 percent blocked, and one was 90 percent blocked. So I'd been walking around, with my heart getting almost no oxygen. Probably the only reason I hadn't dropped dead was because I'd been swimming and my heart was so strong.

I ended up having a quadruple bypass that very day. There I'd been, standing in line to get on an airplane at 11:55, and by 7:30 that night, I was out of surgery. My doctor said that if I'd gotten on that airplane, I'd be dead. If I hadn't come into the ER, I'd be dead. The only thing he said I should've done differently was called an ambulance instead of having my husband drive me to the hospital. So from now on, I won't hesitate a minute to call an ambulance for my friends or for myself.

I got out of the hospital five days later. And you know what? I ended up having a wonderful summer—one of the best of my life—because everybody, all my family members who live here in Hawaii, all my friends, camped out at my house. And everyone was there to take care of me. They'd bring dinner up and we'd all eat together. It was such a pleasure. Everyone was so connected, so present. It was a magical time.

Since then, I've stopped eating cheese, which was my favorite food. I've started walking, and now I walk twenty-five miles a week. I want to get back to swimming, but I'm not supposed to do that for another four months because it takes so long for the sternum to heal from open-heart surgery. Sometimes my chest still hurts, and it's been more than a year. I take my meds and watch my weight, though I need to lose about fifteen pounds. I also get my heart tested regularly. Because of me, so do all my friends and family.

I don't regret at all what happened. On the contrary, I'm very grateful for the experiences my heart event brought me.

Understanding your heart is really, really important. I was a little overweight, but my heart disease was mostly due to genetics and stress. So now I really have to manage my stress. I'm back at work full-time, but I've started a new business, which isn't as stressful.

I really want you women to know that you can't escape your genes. Your heart is your heart, and you are who you are. But that having been said, your family history isn't always as obvious as you might think. The heart disease in my mom's family showed up in her brother and all his kids but not in my mom. So I never considered it genetic. You really have to expand your idea of where your genes come from. I never thought heart disease would get to me. But I have lots of people in my life who love me, a big extended family, including grandchildren, and that's what matters most.

I come from a clan of Sephardic Jews; I call us "Armani Jews" because of our endless joy in celebrating and dressing up. We are a community that shows up for one another and loves to give to one another. We are very traditional, religious, and sometimes even borderline superstitious. We do everything in groups: three hundred strong at a Sunday barbecue, a thousand and counting at a funeral, forty plus at a holiday dinner. My clan also gives new meaning to the terms *lack of boundaries* and *codependency.* But they are also *always* there in numbers in a pinch. We are the original reality-TV show, but then, perhaps one could say that about all families. Ours is the one in Jewish Technicolor.

But there are disadvantages to growing up so closely knitted. And in my clan, the primary one is constant scrutiny—a ticker tape that runs 24/7, indicating the high points and sell points of all whom they encounter. Everyone where I grew up knows everyone else's business. Provocative comments about people's lives spice our conversations like the cumin and cinnamon used in our delicacies. One is judged not only by who one is as an individual but by who one's parents and grandparents are, how much money one has, how one's decorated one's house, how one serves one's guests, and who one's kids marry. If you don't make waves, you can remain a part of everything until you die, and when you do, everyone will show up at your funeral and speak wonderful tomes about you. But in this community, if you make waves, they become a tsunami. I adore my family and community with all my heart, but boy, have we given one another some angina over the years.

The Heart Truth

**Women with a family history of heart disease are two
to three times more likely to experience advanced
atherosclerosis, or hardening of the arteries,
than women with no family history.**

—JOHNS HOPKINS UNIVERSITY SCHOOL OF MEDICINE, 2005

As I said, I was considered the black sheep of the family. Rather than settling down a block from my parents, marrying, and having kids, as I was expected to do, I chose to move away and become a career woman. Where I grew up, "career" wasn't on the list of female life options. "She doesn't want to get married?" was both a question and a way of implying that my parents had done something wrong in rearing me. But I just knew deep in my gut that I could not live the life mapped out so clearly for me by my clan. I had to get out before it was too late. I would suffocate living next door to everyone I knew, never meeting a stranger in the course of a day, only being thought of as somebody's mother or someone's wife. I had to leave because that's who I am. I had no choice, really. And so I made waves by living out of wedlock, living in New York City and then traveling through Europe, starting my own businesses, dancing to my own tune. I always thought it was just too much for my family to handle. But now it seems it was really too much for me to handle.

♡ *The word* no *has a body chemistry, linking women with their heart disease.*

As a result, family gatherings sometimes became claustrophobic experiences. My dramatic life was always the focus when I returned home for a visit, and it was intense. Who would react to what? I never knew. What bomb would I set off when all the family members were in attendance? What mess would I leave behind for my parents to clean up after I was gone? So many!

The Heart Truth

A heart attack occurs on many levels. Look deeper into the reasons: your family history of the disease, your ways of coping with stress, your personal history of health, diet, exercise, smoking, and heartbreak.

—DR. JESSE HANLEY

Not living out the story of the clan breaks many hearts: The grandmother blames the mother, the mother blames the daughter, and so it goes. In my case, the pull between being part of the clan and being separate from it was enormous, the clan's disappointment in me even greater. And it's not as though they kept it a secret. They let me know how they felt as many times and in as many ways as they could. Who needs genes? Guilt, which causes stress, which causes plaque to build up in the arteries, was yet another connection between my illness and me.

The Heart Truth

Stress can play a bigger role in the development of heart disease than butter.

—DR. JESSE HANLEY

In later years, I learned to bring my successes home like others brought home their grandchildren: I won the DeBeers Award for jewelry I'd designed at age twenty-four; I'd opened three gift stores by the time I turned twenty-eight; I was in magazines and on TV; I was a designer; I was this, I was that. Yet it was hard to keep up with my brothers' children and the other grandchildren and cousins as they grew up and started talking. They were real and tangible, and a legacy my family counted on. So I'd whip out stories from my quasi-celebrity life, peppering the climaxes with tidbits from Farrah Fawcett, Barbra Streisand, Cher, Christie Brinkley, and Donna Karan. The family ate these up like the sweet date cookies and rosewater pudding my gramma prepared for dessert, making them forget what a shame it was that I wasn't married and hadn't chosen the life they'd chosen for me. Sometimes I could forget, too. I knew the secret was to leave them wanting more.

———————

Today, I like to ask women I meet, "What happened at the dinner table when you were growing up?" That's because the dinner table is the place where most families define themselves, and, hence, where the stories of who we are get played out. This is where we most often learn our emotional patterns and get physically as well as psychologically nourished . . . or not. Chances are that your family roots go deeper than you'd ever have imagined. We are impacted not just by genetic factors but also by the everyday habits we grew up with, particularly at the table—whether they be drinking, smoking, overeating, gambling, criticizing, maligning, ignoring, laughing, supporting, sharing, or loving.

There's no need to feel ashamed: These patterns are a part of the fabric that weave your personality. We cannot escape where we come from, no matter what geographic or cosmetic makeovers we attempt to give ourselves. Instead, we need to realize that by exploring and understanding our family roots, following them into the deepest places inside ourselves, we can trace a map of our lives. You can change and overcome many things, but it is by blood and blood alone that lives are saved and lives are lost.

♡ *Forgive all you can—especially yourself.*

I bought my mother a gift once, many years ago, a pillow that had sewn into it these words: "Mirror, mirror, on the wall, I am my mother after all." But only after my heart event could I fully accept that and embrace it as the truth.

Heart Song

GLORIA SERURE, *Pamela's mother,*
Long Branch, New Jersey

I called my home "the movers and shakers house." That's what life felt like with all the excitement and drama provided by me, my husband, and our two kids, Pamela and Teddy. Pamela, my firstborn, was an Energizer bunny. She was vibrant, funny, animated, charming, and personable. She stopped only if we sat on her or if she fell ill or went to sleep. She had enormous curiosity about everything, and she was racing to experience it all. Fast and faster were her only two speeds. In addition, she had an independent spirit. By the time she was eighteen, she was living on her own, which wasn't done in our community. But Pamela had her own ideas about how she would live her life.

The sixties, seventies, and eighties were a remarkable career time for Pamela. Getting married and having a family wasn't what called her. She turned her ideas into successful products and grew businesses. Even when she was exhausted, her indomitable spirit didn't let her stop. I often asked, "Pamela, when are you going to catch up to your physical being?"

Eventually, she did reach a place where she no longer wanted to live in Manhattan and work as a marketing executive. So she moved to the Hamptons and began exploring an alternative, healthy lifestyle. That lifestyle became the inspiration to create a juice business. Get Juiced was the talk of the town. Suddenly, Pamela was leading juice retreats to Bali and had a best-selling book. But with all the concentration she devoted to health for others, she neglected her own.

After Pamela finished a worldwide book tour that included endless TV and radio interviews, I finally saw her low-battery light flashing for the first time. Reality had set in, but we had no idea what was coming.

No parent could or should ever be prepared for what happened next. It was Jewish holiday time and, as usual, the whole family got together to celebrate. Pamela had just moved to L.A. a few months prior, but she came home to New York to spend a few days with us. We were thrilled. During her whole time at home, she complained of burning in her chest and diagnosed herself with pneumonia. Now, almost every year of her life she would get sick on these holidays, so I must admit I was a little deaf to it. I did, however, eventually take her to meet with my husband's doctor, a heart and lung specialist, even though we much rather would've been shopping, talking, and running around having fun.

After taking an hour of our precious little time together, the doctor appeared and said, "Pamela is experiencing *angina*." We—in complete unison for the first time in our lives—said, "That's impossible!" He wanted her to check into the hospital. We refused. After all, I've had angina for over twenty-five years, and there's nothing wrong with me. Finally, I felt as though I could protect my firstborn with my strength. So he gave her some nitro, made her sign a waiver saying she wouldn't sue him if she died, and off we went.

When we got home, Pamela collapsed on the bed to take a nap—another first. At last, we are all together and the holidays were great. Pamela left a day later. I sent her off, saying, "Don't worry. After a few days in California, you'll be fine. Check it out when you get there and let us know." But Pamela told me that she experienced that burning sensation again on the flight back to L.A., and it puzzled me. At least I knew that she would now follow up.

The phone rang as I was setting the table for the highest of holy holidays, the Day of Atonement. I picked up, and there was Pamela on the line, saying she would need open-heart surgery in two days. "No, it's impossible," I said. "I can't believe it. We'll be there tonight. How can we be there tonight? Okay, then, tomorrow night. Of course we'll be there. Darling, you are going to be fine. Mommy says don't worry."

The next picture in my head is of my daughter being wheeled through the hospital halls, about to be cut open. I clutched a feather boa I'd brought to wrap her in afterward, knowing how she would laugh. I never believed I could lose her. The severity was still unfathomable. Triple bypass? My husband and I couldn't register the information, even as we sat through the six hours it took to complete the surgery. How could I have protected my daughter from this disease, which I gave to her? I wondered. She got it simply because we share the same blood.

I never realized the toll that heart disease would take on Pamela—physically, emotionally, and spiritually. The damage it did to her beliefs and her body was extensive. She was violated, scarred, and sick—everything she never could have imagined for herself. And she didn't even know the half of it yet. Over the next few weeks, I watched her be the trooper I have always known her to be, but she was putting on a show for her father and me, and we knew it. We had to leave to allow her time to heal.

Eventually, Pamela started to look for cures, for reasons why other women had heart disease, and these she found. She let everything else slip away as she immersed herself in her heart and her healing. So like my little Energizer bunny . . . And now here comes another book, one with valid warning, one with soulful admissions, one with truth for all women.

Thank you, God, for giving Pamela a mind that has helped heal her body and soul. Writing this book lifted her spirits back into the land of possibilities. Knowing my daughter as I do, I am not surprised to see that she has landed safely and healthfully into her new life. She continues to dazzle. She will inspire all those whom she is able to with her joie de vivre, and she will keep on going.

HEALING THE HEART

Prevention of Heart Disease in Women

By Jane Farhi, M.D., cardiologist at Mount Sinai Medical Center

More women (6.9 million) than men (6.7 million) have heart disease. So why on *Desperate Housewives*—the nation's most watched television show, a show that's for and about women—was the character who died of a heart attack a man? Was it a throwback to 1950s thinking, when all the studies and health initiatives were directed at men? Or do the writers of *Desperate Housewives* think that they know their demographics, which reveal (according to the Framingham Heart Study and the Chicago Heart Detection Program) that women under forty-five rarely die of heart attacks?

Either way, I worry that the writers of the show fell prey to a common misconception among Americans today: that women need not worry about coronary artery disease; that heart disease has always been and continues to be a men's disease. This is not the case. Sixty-five is the new forty-five, and by the age of sixty-five, more women than men have heart attacks. Not only is coronary artery disease the leading killer of women, but 25 percent die suddenly, without warning or any prior symptoms of heart disease. One-third of all heart attacks are silent.

How do we approach a disease that can be both silent and deadly? The Framingham Heart Study followed thousands of people for forty-four years, and their children for twenty years. The researchers developed a risk-factor score that has been used to divide asymptomatic, nondiabetic individuals with no overt signs of heart disease into three risk categories: low, intermediate, and high. Doctors can use this data to estimate your risk of having a coronary event in the next ten years. The risk factors that the

Framingham investigators found most significant were age, high blood pressure, total cholesterol, HDL cholesterol, and smoking. For example, a fifty-nine-year-old woman whose cholesterol level is 240, with an HDL—that's the good cholesterol—of 48, smokes, and has blood pressure of 140/80 will find that she has a 14 percent risk of having a heart attack or dying from cardiovascular disease in the next ten years.

It's important to note that the Framingham study did not investigate the following important risk factors: diabetes (because doctors assume you have coronary disease if you have diabetes); early family history; obesity; sedentary lifestyle; history of drug use, particularly cocaine; or stress. It also did not include novel risk factors, such as the use of Vioxx or hormone-replacement therapy.

If you are at high risk—that is, greater than 20 percent risk of a heart attack in the next ten years—you should consult your doctor about aggressive risk-factor reduction. This includes, number one, taking aspirin daily. You may have read on the front page of the *New York Times* that an aspirin a day is *not* recommended for women. That's true for younger women, but here's the fine print: The Nurses' Health Study found that an aspirin a day for women over fifty actually did reduce coronary events by over 20 percent. And the average age of the women in the study was fifty-four. Remember, women get heart disease a decade later than men, so if the average age of women had been sixty-five instead of fifty-four, we could have expected to see even greater benefits, probably closer to a 50 percent reduction in heart attacks, as with men.

The second intervention concerns lowering your cholesterol levels. This has been shown to be just as effective for women as men. You should know your cholesterol levels. An ideal cholesterol profile would be an LDL under 100 and an HDL above 50. LDL is the bad cholesterol, and HDL is the good cholesterol. You can lower your cholesterol levels with medications, and also by controlling your diet. Most importantly, concentrate on eating foods low in cholesterol and saturated fat and high in fiber. Maintaining a healthy weight (waist measurement of no more than thirty-five inches) and exercising regularly (at least thirty minutes most days of the week) will also help naturally lower cholesterol levels.

Third, lower your blood pressure. Though 140/90 is still considered the upper limits of normal, an ideal blood pressure is below 120/80. In fact, recent studies show that we should be talking about prehypertension, which has increased risks similar to those of hypertension, when your systolic blood pressure is between 120 and 140. You can lower your blood pressure with medications, and also by consuming a diet low in salt and rich in fresh fruits and vegetables. People with high blood pressure also should not consume much alcohol (no more than two drinks per day). As with reducing cholesterol levels, you can lower blood pressure by managing your weight and exercising regularly.

If you are in the intermediate risk group, meaning your Framingham score lies between 10 and 20 percent, then you should have screening tests to help better define your risk. These include a test to measure C-reactive protein, which is an indicator of inflammation; a test to determine levels of homocystine and other markers of coagulation; and an ultrafast CT scan, which measures calcium in the coronary arteries and can actually show plaque. A calcium score of over eighty indicates significant coronary disease.

If you're in the low-risk group, you're probably like the women on *Desperate Housewives*. Except for the stress in their everyday lives, they are models of heart-healthy living. They're thin, they jog, they drink in moderation, and they're always chomping on celery sticks. As long as they don't have any other risk factors (such as genetic ones), they may have years of heartache from men, but the probability is they won't have a heart attack—at least not until they're much older.

But regardless of your risk category, both men and women need to pay attention to this silent and deadly killer in our midst. If only Bree had taken her husband's chest pain seriously and gotten him to the hospital sooner, he probably would have survived for another season.

Heart On

My Cure Anything Chicken Soup

For years and years, chicken soup has seen me through colds and the flu, bitter winters, deep depressions, and, of course, heart trouble. I believe chicken soup is the best companion for any illness, but it's especially healing for heart disease. It's the perfect healing combination, rich in nutrients from vegetables, protein, and love; it's filling while not fattening; and mostly it's nurturing for both heart and soul.

Most recipes for chicken soup are pretty similar. But I've been subtly perfecting mine for decades, adding and subtracting flavors. And I firmly believe that I now have the best recipe.

The Best Chicken Soup on Earth

a few tsp. of extra virgin olive oil

2 leeks or 1 medium-size onion

2 large organic carrots

2 large ribs of celery

1½ tbsp. thyme

2 tbsp. coarse salt (sea salt works best)

2 sprinkles black pepper

2 split chicken breasts (organic is best—the taste and quality will be reflected in your soup and in your body)

2 8-oz. cans or boxes of
chicken broth
1½ quarts of water
a handful of fresh parsley,
chopped

a bunch of fresh dill,
chopped
½ cup uncooked brown rice
(optional)

1 | Take a soup pot, coat the bottom with the olive oil, and place over low heat. Slice leeks, carrots, and celery into little disk shapes. Throw them into heated oil with gusto and sauté for 6 to 8 minutes. Add thyme, salt, and pepper.

2 | Rinse the chicken and place in the pot, then create a blessing for all these ingredients. Sauté for 2 minutes. Add broth and about ½ to 1 quart of water, determining for yourself how thin or thick you'd like your soup to be. Praise the chopped parsley, dill, and rice as they enter the pot. You can add other flavors, such as slices of ginger in the winter, cayenne pepper if you like it spicy, or whole-grain noodles instead of rice.

3 | Put on some music. Cook for 2 hours over medium heat, stirring occasionally and acknowledging the good job the soup is doing (soups love to get compliments while they're brewing).

4 | Remove chicken and let cool, then debone. Throw the well-tended pieces of chicken back into the soup and stir, allowing chicken to warm in the broth. Serve with wonderful whole-grain bread and a small salad. Accompany with a delicious glass of cabernet if desired.

♡ *Food should always be served from the heart, with love.*

Heart Song

ELIZABETH O.-F., *Irvington, New York*

When I was thirty-nine years old, I started to feel poorly. I'd get tired much more easily, feel anxious, and sometimes be short of breath. It turns out these are all classic symptoms of heart disease, but I had no idea whatsoever that what I was experiencing was related to my heart. First of all, the symptoms came on very gradually. This disease is insidious. Second, I did not fit the profile at all. I was young, active, and a very healthy eater. I was never a smoker or a drinker. And I'd practiced yoga and meditation for years. What I did have were five-year-old twins and a teaching job at a university in New York City. So I figured my body was just responding to being under too much stress.

The problem was that the symptoms didn't get any better even when I did the right things to relieve stress. I adjusted my schedule so that I worked fewer hours and had to commute into the city less often, and I went to bed earlier, but nothing changed. In fact, I got worse. I started having what I thought were anxiety attacks, heart pounding and sweat dripping. And I'd get these crazy dizzy spells. When I started having trouble walking up the stairs—which I'd had no trouble climbing up an down when I was pregnant with my twins—my husband insisted that I see a doctor.

My general practitioner listened to my story and agreed that I was probably suffering from stress, but he wanted to run some tests anyway. They were inconclusive. So he said, "Let's just wait and see. Pay attention to how you're feeling." I thought maybe I should exercise more, so I started running and doing more yoga. I only got dizzier, more lethargic, and breathless. Sometimes I had to grab hold of the countertop just to stand up.

Eventually, I went back to the doctor, and he sent me to a cardiologist. The cardiologist's tests were also inconclusive. Plus, I didn't have any stabbing or radiating pains, none of the classic stuff. So we still didn't suspect heart disease.

Three months later, my heart was packing up and getting ready to leave. We'd been playing our game of hide-and-seek for long enough. The heart symptoms kicked in full force. I started having palpitations and irregular heartbeats. My cardiologist was now convinced that something was wrong with my heart, though he couldn't figure out what or why. The tests still weren't revealing anything.

Now, I really applaud this doctor, because he did not let his ego stand in the way. Eventually, he admitted that he couldn't figure it out, and he referred me to a pediatric cardiologist. I was thinking, A children's heart doctor? You've got to be kidding me! But my doctor explained why. "First of all, he's brilliant. Second, he is very familiar with unusual, atypical heart conditions and defects because he delivers newborn babies who come into the world with bizarre conditions. Your heart problem could be a congenital defect. Please just go. It's worth a shot."

So I went to see this pediatric specialist in a sort of tongue-in-cheek manner, thinking of it as a joke. But I tell you, the moment I met this man, I recognized what an incredible human being he was. He spoke to me about my condition, looked over my files, did a few simple X rays and CT scans, and within thirty minutes delivered a diagnosis. "I got it!" he exclaimed. "Your heart is failing and you need open-heart surgery."

"What are you talking about?" I replied. I literally could not believe my ears. "I've been coming in for over a year! I've had all these tests! I'm a total health nut!"

He said, "Look, lady, you're dying. Your valve is

leaking terribly. Your heart is working too hard. If you don't fix this soon, you will die."

I was stunned. This whole time I'd thought, This cannot be heart disease. I'm just not the classic candidate. Even now I can't believe it. I knew that there was a family history there, but I'd tried so hard to make my life better that I really thought heart disease would skip me. I did not have the lifestyle my relatives did. My father had died of a heart attack, as had his father, but they'd eaten whatever they wanted and hadn't exercised. Not only that—I had three older siblings who lived more stressful lives than I did and ate terrible food, and yet none of them had heart disease. How could this possibly have happened to me, the healthy one? I wondered.

But what could I do? I was dying. So in early January, I had my open-heart surgery. I was fortunate enough to have a doctor who's called "Golden Hands" because he's such a skilled surgeon. But I think it's more than that. He doesn't bring his ego into the operating room. He says, "This is the work of God," and he performs his surgery by adhering closely to his faith. This man has never lost a patient.

After the surgery, Golden Hands explained to me that I'd had a hole in my heart. Maybe it had been there since childhood, or maybe I'd gotten it later on—we'll never know which. Apparently, children who are born with this defect rarely live past the age of thirteen. So I felt very blessed. The doctor told me that my healthy habits had probably saved my life. That made me feel a little better about the fact that my chest had been ripped open and now scowled with angry scars like a warrior. It made me feel a little better about the fact that my kids had lost their innocence while watching their mother fall so ill.

During the recovery process, I struggled a lot with depression. I felt so ashamed. But I came out the other side a more daring—and, dare I say, better—person. The experience forced me to reevaluate my entire life, and I concluded that I wanted to make some changes. I left my marriage, which wasn't allowing me to grow into the person I wanted to be. I left my university job, which felt too constricting, and got a real estate license. I took my children to visit our homeland, Nigeria. I've become involved with the American Heart Association, helping other women deal with their heart disease.

Here's what I want to say to you: You have to take giant steps, because this is the only life you have. You must be courageous.

4.

THE BOOK
IS SEALED

And the day came when the risk to remain tight in a bud was
more painful than the risk it took to blossom.

—ANAÏS NIN

I'm wrapped in a silver Mylar blanket. I died and have
been reincarnated as a baked potato? I can barely breathe
and my friend K.T. is standing over me. My mouth tastes
like I just drank a mercury martini. What is that thing
squashed down my throat? A Day-Glo plastic ribbed tube
that looks like something out of a George Lucas film. It's suf-
focating me. Two more tubes sprout out of my stomach like
an alien birthing itself. A gaggle more wind in and out of
God knows where on my body. Machines around me beep
on and off, flashing red neon numbers. I feel as though I am
watching my share price plummet on a ticker tape—a bad
day for Pamela stock on the Dow-Jones average.

As I slowly regain consciousness, I hazily recall that I've

just had open-heart surgery. That's why my hospital bed is burning hot: My aluminum foil wrap is designed for cooking, not for lounging. I drip pools of sweat, as if I were in one of my detoxes. If only that were true. I might be hermetically sealed, except that I can still see and hear and smell. I want to vomit, but how? Into the tube I'm choking on? And worst of all, it seems that no one is as upset about this as I am.

The Heart Truth

Women are twice as likely to die from heart attacks as men. Men face a 5 to 6 percent chance of dying after a heart attack; for women, the likelihood of death is 11 to 12 percent.

—AHA, 2005

Nurses on both sides of me calmly, implacably touch, adjust, and monitor the situation. One comes in and puts a phone to my ear. She says it's my sister. When did I get a sister? I'm too tired to argue. I can't say hello; all I can muster is a grunt. How am I supposed to talk with a tube shoved down my throat? The nurse whispers, "It's okay. Just make any sound." She says my sister really needs to know that I'm okay. Then I hear the voice on the other end of the line. My dear friend Donna Karan has convinced the nurses that she is my sister so that she can find out for herself how I'm doing. Most people know Donna Karan as a famous fashion designer. She's complimented throughout the world because of the beauty of her designs, and for the way they make women feel uplifted, sexy, and empowered. Putting all that aside, the way I know her best is as an *anam cara,* a soul friend. And I believe that what she's really about is her big heart. I moan on the receiver and she gets that I'm alive, sort of.

♡ *When you've got heart disease, love is not all you need. You also need financial security, or at least great health insurance, knowledgeable and compassionate doctors, faith, and courage. But love is a great starting point. Don't underestimate how much the love and prayers of your friends and family can help you heal.*

The last twenty-four hours are a blur. I only remember waving to my parents and friends with the back of my hand as the nurses wheeled me through the double doors, down the hallway of Who Knows. I remember my father's face pressed against the windows of the OR, tears rolling down his cheeks. I remember asking God if it was Her will that I return to be on *Oprah* or something like that and do some good for the sake of other women. I also thought I should have let myself have some ice cream. With that thought to comfort me, a peace took over and I was out, into another life.

Then I recall the dream I had the night before. I was sitting on a chair in a room, when Celine Dion came in wearing a bright red dress and sat across from me. She started singing, "My Heart Will Go On," and when she finished she got up and left. That was a consoling dream, the kind you need to help you get to the other side of something so painful.

Heart Song

ANITA F., *Milwaukee, Wisconsin*

Three months before my first heart attack, I went to my doctor and complained like crazy about how exhausted I was. I told him I felt bad all the time. He took one look at me and said, "Anita, you're fat, you're fifty, and you're working too much. What do you expect?" So I went home and cried and felt horrible about myself, but that was that.

Time passed. . . . Now it was December, and I was on my way to a holiday party. I got down to the car, and I started feeling like I couldn't breathe. I was coughing to clear my throat, desperately trying to get more air. This was coming out of nowhere. So I got frightened, and since I had my cell phone with me, I called 911.

A short time later, the fire department showed up.

Four strapping young firefighters came walking over and took my blood pressure, which was really high. I felt so sick. My pulse was 140. They looked at me sitting there, barely able to breathe, feeling worse than I've ever felt in all my life, and told me that because I didn't have any chest pain, I was fine. I had the flu. Then they told me that it would cost three hundred dollars for them to take me two blocks to the hospital, so I should just go home and relax. They said, "This isn't life-threatening." I said, "That's okay, I have insurance. I want to go to the hospital." But they kept talking me out of getting treatment. So eventually I said, "Go away."

I thought about going to bed, but something kept nagging at me. I just knew that I had to get to the hospital. So I very slowly made my way to my car and drove the two blocks there. The parking lot for the ER was full, so I parked about a block away. And very slowly, two steps at a time, huffing and puffing every step, I started to make my way to the entrance. When I got to the circular driveway for the ER, two nurses who (ironically) were outside smoking saw me and realized what bad shape I was in. So they lifted me past the check-in desk and started yelling for a doctor.

Once I was in the ER, they ran a bunch of tests. These revealed that I had pneumonia and was suffering a heart attack. I was frightened. I was thinking,

How could this be? I'm too young. Well, there was no arguing with what was happening. It was surreal, especially after the whole incident with the firefighters. They'd left me feeling ridiculous, like I was being a baby, wanting to go to the hospital. Were they ever wrong!

I didn't call anyone that night. I think I needed time to adjust to what I'd been told. I'd had a heart attack in my early fifties, and it had been a bad one. I had pneumonia. And I needed open-heart surgery. I was just so stunned. Later, when I did tell my parents, they were not amused. I remember trying to explain that I hadn't wanted to scare them. I felt like somebody had pulled the rug out from under me and I couldn't catch myself. I felt like I was falling and falling. . . .

I was in the ICU for a week, because they couldn't do the heart surgery until my pneumonia had cleared up. There was every chance that I would not even make it to the surgery. A priest even gave me last rites. But I did make it. And I made it through the surgery. That's life-altering stuff.

Today, I feel better and happier than I have in years. It's really, really true. I never thought that I would be grateful to have had a heart attack. But my life was not going the way it should've been going. I was working too much, I was exhausted, and I didn't feel good. I wasn't enjoying myself at all. I have turned that around enough so that now life has its rough moments, but there are lots of wonderful things that I enjoy and look forward to. For instance, I'm just so excited to get up in the morning and work out. If you'd told me two years ago that I was going to be addicted to exercise, I would've said, "You're nuts!" But now if I don't go, I feel like I'm missing something.

Also, I took a class in rehab called Freeze Frame. It's a mini meditation session. What they've found is that feeling sincere gratitude can actually make your heart rate slow and your blood pressure go down. So I learned this technique where you focus on your heart, like you're breathing through your heart, and think of something that you're truly grateful for. And I do feel grateful. I have wonderful family and friends. I've had some of the best doctors anyone could hope for. I'm very lucky, truly blessed. So I do these mini meditations for two minutes at my desk, five times a day. It's amazing how well it works. I have the same job, but I handle it so differently. Even my archnemesis can't get to me anymore. I have a different attitude. People are amazed at how I laugh at things that used to make me tear my hair out. Instead of getting upset if something I do doesn't work out, I tell myself, Okay, I made a mistake. I'll learn from it and move on. You can't beat yourself up all the time. I've always been really tough on myself. I'm grateful that I don't have that reaction anymore.

Since my open-heart surgery, I've learned to take the time to enjoy things. Where I live, very close to Lake Michigan, there are mornings when the sun is coming up and the sky turns these amazing colors. And I'm just so excited to be able to see these things.

The hours pass, nonexistent and agonizingly present at the same time, just like my body. I am pure pain. Everything hurts, especially my chest. Finally—minutes, hours, days?—a doctor appears. He yanks the tubes out of my stomach, and I wince. He then pulls the tube from down my throat. That is a huge relief, like breaking a long-endured underwater experience or screaming at a Tina Turner concert. I try to speak, but I feel as though my voice has been taken away. (I won't find out how true that is until months later.)

The surgeon describes what transpired. He says they sawed me open with a real saw, and because I'm so small (oh well, it's all relative, I guess), they broke two of my ribs in the process. Then a clamp pried me open like a newly formed clamshell so they could tend to my arteries. How is it possible that this operation is the most frequently performed in any hospital? It's barbaric! He goes on to say they made a long, snakelike slice up my right leg, from my ankle to above my knee, so they could remove a vein and make it into the two arteries that I needed for the triple bypass. My veins are thin, as most women's are, but they used them anyway. Later on, I will find out that because of this, blood can't flow as freely when I exercise or am under stress. But what else were they going to do, buy some veins on eBay?

He informs me that he made my chest scar a little lower than usual because he heard that Donna Karan is a friend of mine, and he wanted me to be able to comfortably wear her V-necked sweaters again without feeling self-conscious. He actually thought about this? I didn't know doctors consulted with designers on the size of the zippers they put in. Sometimes the truth is hysterical, but this time it was surreal.

The surgeon also says that my heart was held hostage for several hours on the heart and lung machine. What a lovely image; my precious little heart, sitting there, out of time and space, left alone on the Island of Devices that Modern Medicine built. My heart's task was to try and hold on, then reenter without any complications. The surgeon tells me that the second he put mine back, it took. Bam! I was breathing on my own without a hitch, heart and body reunited like estranged lovers. He says he held my heart in his hands; I tell him not many men can say that.

♡ *During open-heart surgery, your doctor will literally hold your heart in his or her hand. Find someone whom you trust, whom you connect with, beforehand if possible.*

97

Experts say that when the heart is removed from the body, it really is like experiencing death. The separation from your heart is what many doctors believe instigates the depression that typically follows open-heart surgery. I know I believe it. Depression came into my life shortly after all this.

It seems that the removal of the heart from the body also causes short- and long-term memory loss, a common side effect of this operation. I wished for months that I could have lost the memory of this event, but no, what I forgot were names of movies, people, and other seemingly important things. I could not download information that I knew I knew, which felt terribly frustrating and confusing. Maybe my brain had decided I no longer needed that stuff. Instead of instant messaging, it was instant deleting. Maybe my subconscious already knew that it was time to make room for new wisdom, new habits, and new insights. Anyway, what choice did I have but to spin it that way?

The Heart Truth

Nearly 40 percent of all female deaths in America occur from cardiovascular disease, which includes heart disease and stroke.

—AHA, 2005

The days in the hospital blended together, from nausea to morphine drips, from changing catheters to the changing of bandages, from the changing of nurses to the ever-present changing of moods. Different hands, different meds, different pains, different meals, none of them good. Every day, answering all sorts of questions with "Yes," "No," "A little," and every day asking "When?" and always "Why? Why? Why?"

♡ *You're on the right path if you don't know what's going to happen next. That's called "a God shot!" Have faith.*

My parents were there. They cried when they were not around me; I could see it in their eyes. They took to behaving like the CNN news scroll. Every fifteen minutes, they would walk into the room and tell me how wonderfully I was doing and how successful the operation had turned out. My chest and my heart disagreed. I felt like I'd just given birth, except there was no baby for us to celebrate. Whenever friends came to visit, trying to cheer me up, I saw the look of horror on their faces. They couldn't be blamed. My bandages oozed, and my chest scar bubbled up pus and other strange bodily secretions. The palette of olives, yellows, and reds that covered my body and reflected the gray-green pallor of the hospital lights hardly matched my fashion sensibilities. My friends, like all people, were drawn to the gore, looking at me with a combination of love, horror, and disbelief. But I have to say that my parents really pulled it off. Thank God for the acting gene that is so dominant in our family. We played along with one another just like we always had. They never left my side except when my friends wanted an audience with me alone. Everyone wanted to hold my hand.

♡ *Hand-holding is the closest we can get to heart-holding.*

Heart Song

ARLENE M., *Quebec, Canada*

My mom, Rae, is a special person. In 1962, when my dad passed away at the age of forty-two, she became a widow with three young children to support. She is no stranger to heart disease; my father suffered from high blood pressure and hardening of the arteries for many years. But sadly, medical technology wasn't as advanced back then as it is today. If so, perhaps my father would have lived longer. Anyway, my mother raised her children with good morals and values, even though she had to do it alone.

Then in 1989, on a monthlong vacation to Florida, my mother wasn't feeling well. The doctor diagnosed her condition as atrial fibrillation—an irregular heartbeat. Rae was slim, watched her diet, and was an avid walker, so she was surprised to hear she had a problem with her heart.

So began her journey into the world of tests, cardiologists, and medications. Through all this, Rae never complained, and as always, she looked so glamorous (much more than I did)! Her condition worsened a few years later. Eventually, she changed cardiologists (thanks to my constant nagging), and she had a pacemaker implanted in 1992. Unfortunately, she developed congestive heart failure and dilated cardiomyopathy—her heart was weakened and could not pump enough blood. Today, she sees a cardiologist regularly to monitor her condition and takes a veritable buffet of medications each day. This for a woman who rarely took a Tylenol in her entire life!

Rae is seventy-seven years young, and to see her, you would never know she has heart disease. She drives, cooks great meals, and goes about her everyday chores to the best of her ability. She lives with a wonderful man, who is very attentive to her needs and understands her limitations. But she tires easily and can't walk far without becoming breathless. Years ago, I couldn't keep up with her on our walks together, so it saddens me to see this change in her. Yet I try really hard to accept her illness and I am upbeat when we visit or talk on the phone, as is she.

It's not easy to watch a loved one battle an illness like heart disease. I worry and pray for Rae a lot. But I also try to feel grateful for the fact that I have such a wonderful mother in the first place. She's got a heart of gold; I just wish it were in better shape.

Three times a day, I shuffled down the Maalox Hall of Fame, saying hello to my fellow heart mates. No one but me was under sixty-five, so each day (given what the memories of heart patients sixty and over are inclined to do), I heard the same thing over and over again: "What is a young woman like you doing here for an operation like this?" This seemed to be the most frequently asked question about me, replacing the previous FAQ, "So when are you going to get married?"

The doctors seemed to feel the same way. I was the favorite viewing specimen for the many med students studying cardiovascular disease because I was the best headline their teachers could have ever wished for: HEALTHY WOMAN TAKEN DOWN IN HER PRIME BY HEART DISEASE! That drew crowds.

The Heart Truth

Thirty-five percent of women, versus 18 percent of men, will die within one year of a first recognized heart attack.

—WOMENHEART, 2005

I had a fabulous male nurse, Aaron, whom I adored. He kept me company every night when I couldn't sleep. Sleeping in a hospital is impossible; there is no such thing as sleep or humility when you are a patient. There is fear, there is projection, there is second-guessing, there is denial, and there is rage, but there is no rest. What's more, the meds kept me in a constant state of nausea. So in would come my knight in shining armor to amuse and distract me with a copy of the *Enquirer*. He'd read me the idle celebrity gossip, share hospital stories, and never forget to tell me how well my healing was progressing. I wish more of the doctors would have followed suit.

My progress was measured in only two ways now: bowel movements and breathing. In order to be released, I had to prove that I had mastered both without the assistance of nurses or machines. After years of perfecting these very same skills alone, it was a novelty to have to try so hard—and then to be graded for my performance. One night, Aaron showed up after being summoned by the floor nurse at four o'clock in the morning for my first bowel movement, something I can honestly say I haven't needed a witness or assistant for since I was three. It felt like I was passing a kidney stone—or rather, a toxic torpedo—yet Aaron was thrilled beyond belief. This was my turning point, he said. Where was I turning toward from a bowel movement? The pain of eliminating all those meds and fears and toxins in one big movement proved to be greater than that of having a zipper sewn into my chest. I was sweating and crying and exhausted, partly due to the pain but also in celebration of my freedom, my imminent release into my new, "normal" life. What a dump it was.

The Heart Truth

Forty-six percent of female, versus 22 percent of male, heart attack survivors become disabled from heart failure within six years.

—WOMENHEART, 2005

Then there was the breathing. Three times a day, we played a game in which I had to breathe into a tube containing a ball. Having practiced yoga and meditation for decades, I felt I had perfected the breathing thing. But breathing with broken ribs and a slice down your chest is kind of like doing yoga with a watermelon tied to your back. The object of the game was to get the ball inside up the tube, thereby clearing my lungs of the idle debris that had filled them during the trauma. I was determined to win this one every day, as if there were a free car or trip to Maui as a prize.

What I did win was an upgrade to the Liz Taylor suite. After ICU, this was a palace, complete with dining room, kitchen, and Liz's own assortment of take-out menus from taco to pizza places. Food was the last thing on my mind. Nausea was always first, while walking and moving came second. Night after night, I sipped ginger ale as if it were a vintage bottle of cabernet while sucking and picking the salt off my saltines in an attempt to conquer the unyielding sensation of seasickness. I was lost at sea, miles away from my usual carrot juice and tofu.

May I take a few moments to vent about how bad hospital hygiene products are? The way they feel and smell is beyond my comprehension. Take note: Everything is antibacterial, antifungal, and antisocial. Sometimes you're given a product that is meant to smell like mangoes or coconuts, but the actual odor is lethal for patients with nausea, like me and most others recovering from surgery. For the $150,000 cost of the operation, you'd think they could throw in a gift basket with a few Aveda products!

I had a window off to the side of my bed that I stared out of for hours each day, marveling at how people were moving around, getting in and out of their cars, carrying flowers to the loved ones they were visiting—and doing everyday tasks with such ease. How had I turned into the visited one? How had I become the one immobilized, while others got to run around? How did this little portal become my world?

It was on one of my many sleepless nights that I finally got up the courage to look at myself. Like a novice stripper, I peeled my robe off first one shoulder and then the other and let it drop to the floor in front of the full-length bathroom mirror. I figured Liz must have done this a thousand times, so I was in good company. It was there in my reflection that the new Pamela came into view, the one with all the markings that made her look as if she'd been initiated into some long-lost island tribe, my cashmere skin branded like a new calf.

The Heart Truth

After menopause, women begin to develop and die of heart disease at a rate equal to that of men.

—AHA, 2005

I was trapped day after day in waves of incredible sadness but still could never manage to cry. Not once since the day they told me I had to live by different rules. Not when I was alone at night, not in between visitors, not after they said I would be on medication forever, not even when I caught the first glimpse of my new and very forever scars. Not even one tear.

I tried to think about my future but never got far. I was at the end of the vision that I'd always had for myself. You would think that I would have felt overwhelming gratitude after having survived an ordeal such as this, but to me, life was now a burden. Who asked for twenty more years like this? Who would want it? Who was I to refuse it?

When a woman undergoes heart surgery, she must come to terms with her longing and the way it will be doused. Heart surgery has a particular flavor to it that is never really discussed—the flavor of bittersweet chocolate. You get a bitter truth and a sweet revelation about your life. Caution: A little goes a long way. Naturally, I did not know then what I know now. But I came to see that all my bravado, ego, and past performances meant nothing to the inner workings of my heart. My fears ruled, while my faith faded. In the end, my courage was really just leftover endurance.

♡ *You get a glimpse of a person's true character when all is lost, when the bag of tricks no longer props up the play.*

After I'd spent two weeks in the hospital, the doctors let me leave. My mother and father came to live with me. I was in their custody yet again, only a little more battered and bruised than the newborn they had carried home forty-seven years earlier. I had to take a regimen of medicines to slow my blood down, and the beta-blockers turned me into a slug. I drank soups and teas up the kazoo, morning, afternoon, and night. My friend Miriam sent amazing blends to soothe me, and they did. But each morning, I took a survey by looking around the room, and each day the same question popped out: "What am I supposed to do now?"

There was nowhere to go and nothing to do. I'd never had a moment like that before in my life, and now suddenly I had thousands of them strewn together. Since music has always been my indoor version of nature and has defined so many of the important moments in my life, I felt that I needed to listen to love songs, especially torchy ones. I listened 24/7 to the same mixes, absorbing love and pain into my heart. It was as if it were the first time I could feel this intensely. Could it be true that my clogged arteries had blocked off my feelings as well as my blood? Could it be that this blockage had led me to make choices in my life that I could now change? Music became my words, my emotions, the way I defined time. Music was my background to stare at the life that had fled somewhere between the saw and the scar.

♡ *Time goes slower when you are healing, so you must*
follow. Speeding allows you to overlook those parts of
you that have been hiding for years.

My dear friend Geneen came to care for me. She tended to me better than any nurse ever could have. She was there from the beginning of this saga until the end, because that's just the way she is, and thank Goddess for that. She became the clearing station through which everything and everyone from the other world had to pass. K.T., my parents, various visiting nurses, and even Dr. Hanley took part in the revolving care and love I received. Some days, that was comforting, and some days it became claustrophobic. I felt more like a caged cougar than a princess being waited upon hand and foot.

Friends and business acquaintances called constantly and sent flowers and cards every day, but even as the gifts and tokens for healing multiplied, I struggled to find my voice. It kept getting lower and deeper. Eventually, I asked Geneen to leave a message on my answering machine saying, "Thanks for calling. While I very much appreciate your thoughts and concerns about me, I cannot return your call at this time." I felt like that gave me some freedom. Two weeks later, my parents had to leave. I needed to grieve, and grieving in front of one's parents is not an easy thing to do if you are the one who traditionally enlivened. I could not keep up the charade of getting better when inside I felt as if I were dying.

K.T. sent over a masseuse who sang as she massaged. She thought the combination of music and touch would help me revive. That sounded as normal to me as it probably sounds crazy to most of you. Remember, L.A. has a reputation to keep up. She began to sing me a lullaby as she placed me gently on the table like a newborn. She touched me in soft strokes and sang her heart songs angelically, stroking my scar over and over, until there she found it, the oil well of tears, and opened the floodgates to my sorrow.

I started to sob in waves, like the ones breaking outside my window. I sobbed for past, present, and future pains. I sobbed as though I were mourning someone close to me who had died, and I had begun to realize that someone was me. I sobbed as if I was in the presence of something sacred. I sobbed like I had never let myself sob before. The masseuse read my scars as if they were braille. My body responded to her touch as if I were an instrument and music was the language we could both understand. This kind and unusual stranger brought me home to myself with a love song—one that had been inside me all along.

♡ *Music is a wonderful medicine for the heart: It involves romance, memory, dreams, and movement— all of which are stalled for awhile in recovery.*

HEALING THE HEART

Getting the Treatment You Deserve

By Matthew Budoff, M.D., cardiologist, associate professor at UCLA School of Medicine

Heart disease among women has been on the rise over the last twenty years. Furthermore, it is on the rise relative to men, because the rate of heart disease among men is going down. Today, 38 percent of women, versus 25 percent of men, will die within one year of a first recognized heart attack. Why is this the case? And what can you do about it?

First of all, heart disease is decreasing in men because doctors use cardiac drugs (such as cholesterol-lowering medicines, blood pressure pills, and even aspirin) on them with higher frequency. We are not applying these medicines as aggressively to women, so more women are having cardiac events than men. Second, many heart tests are flawed for women. This is likely due to the fact that most tests were first studied in men. Women comprise only 25 percent of participants in all heart-related studies, and yet there are obvious gender differences in hormone levels, and there is the added factor of breast tissue in women. Finally, women are more likely to present with unusual or nontypical symptoms, such as shortness of breath, rather than chest pain, so doctors sometimes miss their signs of heart disease.

The medical community needs to do its part to improve the ability to diagnose heart disease in women by recognizing the treatment gap, and by remembering to be on the lookout for the disease in women. Women should also do their part to ensure that they are getting the best-possible treatment and are being properly diagnosed by educating themselves. The best way to detect heart disease in women is the ultrafast CT (to look for either calcium or blockage). Find out if this or another test is appropriate for you. Know that treadmill tests do not work well in women, and that nuclear tests expose you to high levels of radiation and also tend to give false readings in women.

Don't let your knowledge that more women than men die of heart disease and stroke every year frighten you; let it empower you. Understand your risk factors for heart disease (family history, obesity, age, diabetes, high cholesterol, high blood pressure, and smoking), realize that you may be at risk, and seek out further evaluation if you are.

HEART ON

Screaming and Shaking

So I am searching for my deeper voice, the one inside me that rises for my screams and shrinks for my whimpers; the voice that's sure of what she knows; the one that drowns out the voice that is frightened and clueless on this new journey. I need this voice now; I need her to help me live the everyday. I should be able to draw on her like water from a well. Instead, I feel abandoned.

With a pen in my hand, I often am dominated by her voice, my muse, who has been with me for so long. Typically, we meet only for as long as it takes to put the words on the page; then we part like lovers after the affair, running back to our normal lives, our regular partners. The wordsmith in me has always waited impatiently for her visits.

But things have changed a great deal since the surgery. I no longer have patience. Our relationship has become tempestuous. There is no room for meandering about the dark holes inside, searching for her. I want her to be available to me—on demand and on target. I fear that impersonators have already taken control. They hold her hostage, trying to keep my neuroses agile.

I first met my voice at age twelve, when a yearning for poetry overtook my body like a religious fervor and carried me into a frenzy of words, pouring images onto pages. I have not been as generous with her as I have with my daughter voice or my ego declarations or my lover's whisper or my big boss bellow. They have been my favored children, the voices that got me the scholarship, the money, the success, the voices that prospered the more I orphaned her. But what was I to do? She wanted to make a poet out of an entrepreneur! It never would have worked. Nevertheless, we continued to meet time and again, always passionately yet always briefly, over the next forty years.

Now that I have been to death's door, I have that different sight. I want to say it as I see it. I want to be more languid with her, this strong partner inside me. I'd like to travel for a while through her deep voice, cavernous with feeling. I want to know who she is. Is she sexy? Earthy? Eccentric? Does she bathe, or shower? Does she cook, or order in? Does she judge, or accept her fate? And is she at peace with popping in and out of my existence? She has been calling on me for years, and yet just when she caught my attention, she hides herself away.

Where are you, deep voice? The diminutive giant goddess that undulates from my tongue onto the page, that makes me strong, that gives me faith. I am looking for you, and I won't rest now until I find you.

Heart Song

CHRISTINE G., *Central Islip, New York*

My story is quite common, with the exception of one thing: my age. I was just twenty-seven when all this happened.

It was March 16, 2005, a Wednesday. I'll never forget that day for the rest of my life. I was at work, doing my normal routine, but I wasn't feeling too well. I'd been to my regular doctor the day before because I was coughing a little and had been experiencing some minor chest pains. She'd said I probably had an upper-respiratory infection, and so she had put me on antibiotics. Usually, these gave me major stomach cramps, so that day I waited until an hour before I was going to get off work to take them. But only twenty minutes after taking the antibiotics, I already had terrible cramps! My boss told me to go ahead and leave.

At that exact moment, I started to sweat profusely, to the point that I had to take one of my shirts off. I felt like I needed to get fresh air because I couldn't catch my breath. So I grabbed my jacket, pocketbook, and keys and started walking briskly down the hall. As soon as I got outside, I collapsed. I fell to my knees, trying desperately to catch one single breath, but I couldn't. I was so scared. I thought I was having some kind of crazy reaction to the antibiotics. Just then, one of my coworkers passed by and saw what kind of condition I was in. He ran to call me an ambulance. (Thank God he wouldn't let me leave! I lived only five minutes from work and would've tried to drive myself home.)

The first official on the scene was a police officer. He gave me oxygen and told me over and over again that I was having an anxiety attack and needed to calm down. At this point not only was I sweating and couldn't breathe; I also had stabbing chest and back pain that would come and go every couple of minutes. I started to think I was dying. I told my colleagues to call my husband, who was working about two hours' driving time away, and my sister-in-law.

When the ambulance finally arrived, the EMTs said the same thing about my having an anxiety attack. Now, I had no idea what anxiety felt like. I'd never been in the hospital before and nothing serious had ever happened to me. But I knew this wasn't psychological. I just knew that something wasn't right! So the ambulance driver took me to a hospital about fifteen minutes away, where my sister-in-law was waiting for me. As soon as they took me out of the ambulance, I told her I thought I was dying. My chest hurt so bad that I still couldn't breathe.

In the ER, the doctors and nurses hooked me up to all sorts of machines and did a bunch of blood tests. They couldn't figure out what was going on. They wanted to know if I took drugs and I said, "No! None!" I kept telling them that I was having massive chest and back pains, and I was obviously experiencing shortness of breath and sweating like crazy. I told them that heart disease runs in my family (my father had triple bypass at forty-seven; my uncle had a heart attack last May). They even hooked me up to the EKG machine about six times within four hours, and my results were completely abnormal. And yet they still didn't diagnose a major heart attack! They were simply in denial because I was so young.

When my parents and husband finally made it to the hospital and saw the poor shape I was in and that the staff was doing nothing for me, they got really upset. My father told them to give me an aspirin, because it sounded like I was having heart problems. Finally, the cardiologist came in. As soon as he hooked me up to the EKG, he figured out what was going on and gave me aspirin and rushed me to St. Francis, a cardiac hospital. It turned out I'd been having a massive heart attack for the past five hours! The staff at St. Francis was waiting for me when I arrived, and they sped me immediately to the OR to have a stent put in. I later found out that my arteries had been 95 percent blocked.

I've only just begun my journey down the long path to recovery. It's been nine weeks now since the surgery. I feel very frightened, but at least I'm alive. I've been doing on-line research to find out about my disease, and that makes me feel better. And I've gotten a ton of support from other women with heart disease in chat rooms on-line (www.heartcenteronline.com—see page 202 for more information).

I now know that the doctors and nurses in the other hospital had no knowledge about heart conditions in younger people. I had every single symptom of heart disease in women. They just did not want to believe that I was having a heart attack, because I was young, athletic, ate well, didn't do drugs, and weighed only 130 pounds naked. But I'm here to tell you that if it can happen to me, it can happen to anyone. So believe your body when it doesn't feel right. Don't let the doctors try to talk you out of it. *You* know best.

5.

THE THREE STOOGES
OF HEALING:

Disbelief, Denial, and Depression

When you give up hope, your heart goes as well.
The heart is the most poetic organ in the body.

—DR. MEHMET OZ

I was so very, very tired. Exhaustion permeated my whole
being—exhaustion from what had just transpired, exhaustion from what had been my life so far. I never slept anymore because I couldn't turn right, left, or onto my belly. I'd
never mastered sleeping on my back and my chest wound
certainly didn't make it comfortable to move any other way.
Pain radiated throughout my body. Days and nights were a
blur. My body felt like pizza dough without the toppings,
flattened and pummeled.

I had a cavernous and excruciatingly painful wound in
the middle of my chest, snaked with a demon of a scar. The

ribs that had been broken during surgery didn't appear to be in any hurry to mend, and my usually high spirits had disappeared, leaving no note to indicate when they'd be showing up again. I felt like a jack-in-the-box, the kind you play with when you're three years old. Pop goes the weasel! The weasel, it turned out, was depression.

The Heart Truth

Depression and the heart are sisters. Depression is a common warning sign of a heart attack, as well as a common consequence of one.

—DR. GALINA MINDLIN

Depression is an insidious and indiscriminate visitor. It doesn't knock, pick a good time to drop by, or wait for an invitation to enter. It doesn't dress in bright colors or crack jokes or ever want to leave. It simply shows up and nestles in like a long-awaited guest, lounging on the sofa. Depression has no single personality trait. It camouflages itself within its host. So you don't know until you have it whether it'll make you eat or sleep too little or too much, cry all the time, or get angry. The only constant is moodiness. It can feel like a heavy down blanket that covers you, but it also can feel like a gossamer nightgown enveloping you for days on end. It can be handled but never thrown off entirely. It permeates like carbon monoxide, deadly and invisible to the eye but always apparent to the heart.

♡ *Depression is measured by its weight, not height, and it's usually heavier than the person carrying it.*

Heart Song

SHARAMI K., *New York, New York*

When I was fifty-one years old, I experienced real depression for the first time in my life. By that, I don't mean I felt sad for a few days or so. It was as though a gray veil was hanging in front of my eyes. I tried to shake the feeling, but when I didn't want to water the plants anymore, I realized that something was really wrong. As a therapist, I knew that I needed help. I started taking an antidepressant for a few months. This treatment helped me change a difficult situation for the better, which changed my need for the meds. So I stopped taking them.

A couple of years after this depressive episode, when I was fifty-three, I began having dizzy spells some mornings. I also noticed a lot of indigestion. I used over-the-counter drugs for heartburn to combat the indigestion. I ate a bigger breakfast for the dizziness, which I thought was related to the hypoglycemia (low blood sugar) I'd suffered from in my youth. When I started to experience shortness of breath going up subway steps or hilly streets, I attributed this to being out of shape. In retrospect, if one of my friends or clients had described these symptoms to me, I would have immediately suggested that she see a physician. But in my own case, I viewed each of the symptoms individually rather than collectively. So often, we don't listen to or help ourselves in the careful, attentive way we would another.

About six months after these feelings began, I had a severe heart attack. It was a Saturday morning in October 2000. I was in my kitchen, talking with a friend, when I got dizzy and almost fell to the floor. My friend helped me sit down and drink a glass of orange juice. About twenty minutes later, I felt better. We had breakfast, my friend left, and I went about my day.

The following Friday, I went to see my primary-care physician for a previously scheduled visit. I mentioned the dizzy spells and indigestion in passing. She did an EKG and shocked me when she said, "My God, you've had a major heart attack." The heart attack had occurred when the largest coronary artery, the left anterior descending (LAD), had become blocked. I was told that 75 percent of people who have that artery obstructed die instantly. I felt how very lucky I was and that clearly, in my language, "it wasn't time." I had more work to do here on this planet.

My physician wanted to know why I hadn't come to see her sooner. I could only answer that it's a woman's issue. Most women don't pay attention to the signals their bodies are sending, but they would pay attention if any of their family members had similar symptoms. Perhaps it is part of the superwoman complex that women have of being able to scale tall buildings and get through everything for everyone in a day.

My new cardiologist ran a battery of cardiac tests, which revealed that I needed bypass surgery. Since only one artery was blocked, I was able to wait several months for the surgery. During that waiting time, my cardiologist kept asking me if I was depressed, saying that depression is common after a heart attack. I would always say no. But then one day, I noticed that gray cloud returning and recognized that I was becoming depressed again. Only this time, the depression felt deeper; it felt like it was in my body, not just my mind. I began to take Celexa daily, which had the remarkable effect of getting rid of the depression rather quickly. I felt emotionally better but still very tired physically. I stayed on Celexa until the day before the heart surgery, then discontinued it to see if I would need it postsurgery.

Actually, after the surgery I felt ecstatically happy to be alive. I said a prayer of gratitude each morning when I awoke and each night before I went to sleep. I valued every day more than I ever had before. My life was fine as I healed from the surgery, and I went back to work. But then four months after the surgery, the depression was back again. It was clear that it was not situational, as my life was wonderful. It was brought about by my heart disease. I went on an antidepressant again and continued to take it for almost two years. I also feel that it took almost two years for me to recover fully from the heart attack and subsequent surgery. When I felt totally like myself again, I decreased and then discontinued my use of the antidepressant. While I no longer take the medication, I am grateful for having had it in my time of need.

Today, my heart is functioning well, and so is my life. In fact, a month ago I was so happy, someone told me an overabundance of joy could hurt my heart. I told him, "Please include that in my eulogy someday."

♡ *Living never wore one out so much as the effort not to live.*

—*Anaïs Nin*

Mine was a virgin depression. Never having suffered a bout of it before, I found it seduced its way into me, making me feel oddly reassured at first. It started with me idly staring out my window for days, not able to be or do much else. I stared at the ocean and the sky until I was blind—blinded to my past, blinded to my dreams, blinded to my new reality, blinded by the sun. I was most assuredly blindsided by the pain, both internal and external. I stared outside so much because I did not want to have to look at what was going on inside me. And yet the more silent I became, the more animated my depression grew. I became sensitive, cranky, teary, bitchy, grouchy, sad, and pessimistic: the Seven Dwarfs rolled into one. Worse yet, I soon discovered that I had no control, no ability to stop it.

They say all you need is a crack to let the light in; Leonard Cohen has a song about that. Well, I had a cavernous and excruciatingly painful hole in the middle of my chest, big enough for a lighthouse beacon, yet still the darkness conquered me.

My depression gave me an entirely new personality. It was low, quiet, and very negative *(quelle surprise)*—all opposites of the old me, what I still thought of as "the real me." This persona had no identity yet. She didn't cook, sleep, shop, or laugh. I didn't even know the simplest things about her, such as what she liked to eat or wear, or how she got things done. But somehow she had *become* me. I, the *über*-foodie, the one who used to stock her refrigerator as if it were wartime, now had lost my appetite for everything. I, who had loved life so much, now seemed able to think only of death. Nothing fit anymore: My clothes were too big; my voice was too low; my body was a mess. I felt as though I was trapped in a carnival fun house, but certainly without any of the fun.

The Heart Truth

Individuals who suffer from depression are four times more likely to have a heart attack than those who aren't depressed.

—NATIONAL INSTITUTE OF MENTAL HEALTH (NIMH), 2001

My illusions about health, happiness, and love lay scattered in a million pieces, like a broken plate on the kitchen floor. My only hope was one day these beautiful bits of mosaic would come together to create an artistic form for my new life. Each day, though, became another foray into a place that had more and more doors but fewer exits, more questions but never any real answers. I would lie in bed every night—so still, opened like a new bride—wanting to be captured. I was waiting for an image, a voice, or a message to tell me what my next steps should be. But nothing and no one came. I started thinking about death all the time—not in terms of committing suicide, but, rather, in the sense that dying felt like the logical next step. That thought both surprised me and left me feeling very agitated.

♡ *Having heart disease is like giving birth or falling in love: You have to be ready for whatever it brings.*

I honestly had no desire to do anything but sip tea, stare at the ocean, and watch *Oprah.* Thank heavens for Oprah; she can lift anyone's spirits. She is definitely Everywoman's soul mate. Her makeovers delighted me, her no-nonsense approach comforted me, and the spiritual moments in which she reflected people's courage to transform themselves inspired me. Unfortunately, *Oprah* occupied only one hour out of twenty-four in a day. Why can't we have her replace the nonstop news on CNN?

Weeks after returning home from the hospital, I felt that I could not tote the wheelbarrow of my depression any longer; I was a one-hundred-pound mule with a five-hundred-pound load. I had no references for the way I felt, no one to confer with about it, no fashion forecasters to tell me what to wear for it, no other women in my age group to call up and cry with over it, no members of support groups that I knew of with whom I could share my story. Here I was, my heart split wide open, and there were no takers. I felt more alone than ever.

♡ *When you feel your path is bleak or that your soul has made a mistake, hold on a little longer. Your real journey is stretching out its course. Time is a stranger where healing is concerned. But in the end, your heart will find its way home.*

I had to go in for postsurgery checkups weekly. All the machines and all the doctors were happy with my progress. We seemed worlds apart in our thinking. The fourth week I went in, when my depression had fully taken over, I finally got an answer. After the testing was complete, the nurse, Susan, closed the door.

"Pamela, how are you really?" she asked. "I mean *really?*" She said "really" as though it were a code word for us to speak honestly.

I replied, "Susan, I am depressed all the time and I can't shake it."

She nodded her head. "Yes, I know. That's what happens."

"What do you mean, 'That's what happens'?" I asked.

"To people who have had open-heart surgery," she replied.

> ## *The Heart Truth*
>
> **While one in twenty American adults experience major depression in a given year, that number rises to one in three for heart attack survivors.**
>
> —NIMH, 2001

"Why is something like this being kept secret? The doctors told me I'd be on the golf course in six weeks. It's already been four weeks and I don't remotely know how or want to play golf!"

Susan smiled and came closer. Softly, she asked if I wanted some meds to help me through this difficult time. She must have done this a thousand times before, and yet she said it in a hushed tone of voice, as if a drug transaction were taking place. "What kind of meds?" I asked, intrigued.

"Antidepressants," she said. "You would only have to take them for a while, just until you feel back to yourself."

"What if I never feel back to myself?" Recently, I'd come to accept this as a distinct possibility.

"You will, don't worry," Susan said soothingly.

"How will I know who my 'self' is anymore, even if she does come back? And if I take these meds, how do I know they won't take me further away from myself?"

Susan put her hand on my shoulder. "Please think about it," she urged. "You don't have to suffer like this."

"Don't you feel that ship has sailed?" I replied.

Susan then suggested an antianxiety drug or some pills to help me sleep. I refused again. I honestly did not want anything to help take the edge off—been there, done that. I said I would give it another two weeks and then reconsider.

Why, after years of popping pills, wouldn't I agree to take some now on the chance of escaping this horrible depression? The answers were:

a. I did not believe in them.
b. They scared me.
c. I liked the depression.
d. All of the above.

Heart Song

RACHEL G., *Boston, Massachusetts*

Ten years ago, when I was forty-six years old, I started feeling fatigued. I'd worked out for twenty years, wasn't overweight, didn't have a cholesterol problem, ate decent foods, and had never smoked, so most of the risk factors for heart disease weren't there. I did experience some discomfort in my forearms from time to time when I was walking up a hill or doing an aerobics class. But I never had any chest pain, so I didn't make the connection to my heart.

This went on for several weeks. Then one day, I had to turn around during a walk and go home because the pain in my arms got so bad. I lay down on the couch, thinking it would get better, but instead, I began to feel worse. Then out of the blue, a picture popped into my head—I really believe in the grace of God, let me tell you. I saw this diagram from a medical book I'd read years and years earlier, a drawing of a man that showed where you might have pain during a coronary event. And I remembered that it showed pain extending down the inner arm. So I thought, Could I possibly be having a heart attack?

I went to see my doctor, and he sent me to a cardiologist, who did a stress test. He saw some irregularities on the EKG, but he wasn't sure if there was anything wrong. So he sent me to the nearest hospital, where I had a catheterization under local anesthesia. When I was done, he came into my room and said, "You need a bypass. You have ninety-five percent blockage. But just a single artery." I was a workaholic, running my own business, always go, go, go. I said, "I can't have a bypass. I have seminars to lead this week!" But my husband, who was in the room with me at the time, looked at me and wept. He had just lost both his parents and his brother at age fifty-three, so he was scared to death. I was not scared at all. I'd had a number of abdominal surgeries for endometriosis, so I was cool and collected.

For my surgery, I went to Mass General, the leading hospital in the area for this type of operation. I had to wait three days for the bypass. It went well, and I only had to stay in the hospital for five days. Then I was anxious to get back to work. I wanted to show everyone that I could bounce back, do everything that I had done before. I wanted to prove that coronary heart disease had nothing to do with me. I wanted people to say, "Isn't Rachel a whiz?"

Recovery was very frustrating because I had to exercise so slowly and methodically. I wanted to run faster, work out harder. I thought, This is ridiculous. But I was my own worst enemy. While I did well taking it easy for the first eight weeks or so, after that I was off to the races. The problem was that I was never okay with the idea of having heart disease. I thought, That's for old people, people who are fat, people who don't work out, and that's not me. Psychologically, I was not very accepting of myself. I wasn't giving myself what you need after you've gone through something like this.

So I went straight back to working round the clock, exercising hard, drinking too much. I wanted so much to be carefree, to do what I wanted. And almost a year to the day later, I wound up in a psychiatric facility. I was clinically depressed. Not only was I ignoring my heart experience but I was also having issues with my mother's psychiatric health and grappling with my own long road of infertility, which had come to an end with a hysterectomy. I was grieving, working like a lunatic, and taking care of both my parents. It was too much responsibility. Any normal person would have said, "No, enough is enough." But it's that woman's side of me, the people pleaser, always wanting to take care of others but not myself. So I wound up spending five days in a lock-down psych hospital. And I needed to be there.

After that, I did a pretty comprehensive stress-management program. In the past, if there was something I didn't want to think about, I'd always dive deeper into work and that would make me feel competent. Through the stress-management program, I learned the value and techniques of meditation. That helped a great deal in my recovery. I believe that meditation can be the answer for someone as stressed-out as I was. Because if you get to that place where meditation takes you, then you're living mindfully, so you'll be more likely to exercise, eat well, set your priorities, and take care of yourself. I still struggle with stress and workaholic tendencies, but if I stop and meditate twenty minutes a day, it really helps. I also started taking antidepressants, which were a great relief.

It's been ten years now since my heart surgery, and there have been a lot of ups and downs. I'll make slow progress, then slip again, then make more progress. I'm still struggling with my need to prove myself through work, be entertaining and smart. But I have a new attitude. What's the point? I ask myself.

I've sung in the church choir ever since. Music really grounds me; it helps me feel more in touch with myself and that which is greater than I am. I don't drink anymore. I'm tired of cooking, so I still struggle with eating well, but my weight is normal because I watch my carb intake. I work out with weights now as well as doing cardio exercise. I do yoga. I take cholesterol-lowering drugs. I do everything that I should do to stave off another cardiac event.

I'd love to tell you that I've arrived. But I haven't. In my own mind, I'm still always trying to prove, trying to prove. I tried even harder after the bypass, and that landed me in a psychiatric facility. And yet at least I've managed to simplify my life. I sold my dad's business. I'm trying to think about working less, maybe dropping to twenty-five hours a week. On one level, I want to have more space and air in my day, but on the other hand, I'm fighting a constant battle with myself because I'm such an urgency addict. "Ooh, I need to go here, I need to go there," I tell myself. Many women do that. I definitely do. I need constant reminders; otherwise, I gravitate toward things for which I'll be reaffirmed and acknowledged. I want people saying, "Isn't she smart? Isn't she great?" It's that ongoing need to please everyone and make everyone think you're so cool. It's a sickness, actually. I know from experience, from my depression and psychotherapy.

It's life or death. I could wind up back there with a heart attack. It could happen. I still have the same genes, and I'm still under a lot of stress. When I hear myself speak like I'm speaking to you now, then it reminds me that I have to change. I have to slow down. But it's a lifelong process, getting your head screwed on straight when it comes to taking care of yourself.

Let me say right here and now that no matter what specific type of heart surgery you have, you will never be the same—not necessarily better or worse, more conscious or less sympathetic, thinner or heavier, as there is really no judgment about who inside you wants to emerge in the end. Part of you *will* emerge, though, whether or not you like her, want her, or think you need her.

I'll say it again: No matter what, *you will never be the*

same. Why can't they (the doctors, the nurses, the Web sites, the healers, the ones who've been through this before) just tell you that? It's a disservice to the soul of a person not to communicate the alienation she will feel once her heart is tampered with. What are they so afraid of, anyway? I mean, it could be very exciting to think, After this surgery, I am going to be different. Great! I needed to be different. What a boost that is, what a bonus to the trauma: the promise of seeing changes in your self. A new self, one who won't bore you, ridicule you, harass you, or even diminish you. One who is up for a change and takes on the challenge willingly. Why not? Why can't they tell you *that* before they dim the lights?

The Heart Truth

Most heart patients with depression do not receive appropriate treatment, because their doctors and care providers tend to miss the diagnosis.

—NIMH, 2001

Well, I'm here to tell you that something really does happen to you once your body is cut open. Whether it's molecular, physiological, or emotional, there *is* a significant change that occurs, and it *is* real. Do not let anyone tell you otherwise. You are the one who experiences the differences inside yourself. As women, we react in body and mind. I mean, when was the last time you heard a man freaking out over his thighs being too heavy? We are different creatures, and— most of the time—neither male nor female doctors can morph themselves into our body experiences. Please honor what you feel. Trust yourself. People who have met you for the limited number of hours it takes to have an operation don't know you or even have the time to know you. Certainly they can't know you the way you know yourself.

♡ *Instinct is that essence of thought untouched by our schemes. When you have heart disease, it's more important than ever to listen to your instinct.*

Since I didn't want to take meds—not that there's anything wrong with antidepressants; they just weren't what I was pulled toward at this point in my healing process—I turned to Dr. Hanley. She proposed a number of ways for me to try to relieve these overwhelmingly dark feelings: herbs, breathing exercises, positive imaging. They ran the gamut of alternative thinking. And they did help, but they did not cure.

So I forced myself to look a little deeper. What makes you *really* happy, Pamela? I asked myself. When no one is looking, what truly satisfies you? What is essential to your life?

It was with that question that all my voices suddenly reappeared and orchestrated a climatic moment. There it was, the kernel that popped, the idea that got a rise out of me, just like an unexpected kiss. The question is always better than the answer. Sitting on my rocker while waiting for *Oprah* to make my day, having a bowl of chicken soup, Sage at my feet, wearing my cashmere sweats—that's when it entered. I heard it distinctly, enunciated perfectly: Do nothing. Do nothing, Pamela.

Never before had I connected with *wanting* to do nothing or thinking that was an answer to anything. I had always wanted to do *more*. More was my significant other. It was now the spring of 1999 and "Do nothing" was going to be my personal way to ring in the new millennium. I had to allow that to be the most intuitive part in answering my call, for I had nothing else to go on.

♡ *Be content to* be *and not* do*, especially while you're*
   healing. Remember the lessons of kindergarten: Play
   for a while, and then nap and have a cookie.

Two pieces out of those hundreds on the floor suddenly began to make sense and come together. In fact, they were a perfect fit. I could stare, write, sip tea, walk Sage, paint, cook, watch movies, sleep, and eventually *heal*. Oh my God! What a concept. I could slowly come into a new rhythm, one that not only would serve my health, myself, my life but would also allow my depression its due. I think this is what most people refer to as balance. I did not opt for the antidepressants; I opted for the "Do nothing" prescription. This was the medicine I could stomach, and so I wrote the script.

The Heart Truth

Depression may make it harder for you to take your meds and follow through on other treatments for heart disease. It can also cause chronic elevation in stress-hormone levels, further damaging your heart. Don't be afraid to diagnose yourself and seek treatment for your depression.

—NIMH, 2001

We heart women need to get rid of the stigma surrounding depression. We really do take everything to heart. That is our birthright as women, and we must live it and sometimes act it out. Why should we be made to feel that there is something wrong with us if we suffer a bout of the blues, especially following such a traumatic event? Why do we think that we have to run away from our depression, mask it, or rename it? Taking medications is definitely the ticket for some, but for others, it can prevent you from venturing in and enjoying the ride. Why is it that we think that sadness is the part to fix in ourselves, while happiness is our true destination? Why do we try to *think* away what we *feel*, when inside we know it has never ever worked that way? I think the Beatles said it best: "Let it be, let it be." Whichever method you choose to assist you, make sure it's yours: your decision, your wish, your nature. It's *your* healing process, after all. It's *your* heart.

HEALING THE HEART

Music, Emotions, and the Heart

By GALINA MINDLIN, M.D., PH.D. in neurophysiology and neuropsychology, assistant clinical professor of psychiatry at Columbia University

Depression, anxiety, and stress all contribute to heart disease. Negative emotional states create a domino effect inside the body: cortisol levels skyrocket, your arteries constrict, your immune system slows down, your heart rate increases, and your blood pressure climbs. Over time, these unhealthy responses take their toll in the form of disease (especially heart disease and cancer) because your body simply cannot bear the stress. The tighter you hold on to your emotions, the more damage you do to your heart. Learning to control your emotions is therefore one of the most crucial keys to a healthy heart. You've got to be able to let go, give up the fight, and take a break.

It is especially important for women with heart disease to mediate their emotional reactions, because their hearts are so vulnerable. Yet as women, we generally rely on our feelings to negotiate our way through life, so this can prove quite a challenging task. Furthermore, women with heart disease tend to have type A personalities, meaning they need to be in control. Yet when they have a heart event, they lose all control. Their response to this lack of control triggers stress, which causes more symptoms to appear, and eventually exacerbates the disease itself.

Whenever there is turmoil or chaos in your life, make an effort to be calm, act calm, and bring calm into your body. Before confronting a known stressor such as a bad boss or a bad marriage, first try to get yourself into the zone—one in which you feel calm, centered, and ready to take on whatever life brings your way. You can accomplish this through meditation, deep breathing, exercising, getting some sunshine and fresh air, reading poetry, giving someone a hug, singing, laughing, or spending time with a pet, among many other options. These activities immediately help counterbalance the effects of stress by relieving tension, quieting the mind, slowing your heart rate, reducing constriction in your blood vessels, and lowering levels of stress hormones.

While many doctors and psychologists overlook this simple method, I highly recommend listening to music.

Music frees the mind and reduces pain. Thousands of years ago, the Greeks and Romans used music as therapy. Today, music has been found helpful in treating heart-related ailments such as high blood pressure, unstable angina, and depression, and in speeding recovery from surgery. Clinical trials demonstrate that women and men who listen to music during operations have a much more positive outlook regarding the experience.

There is no stigma associated with listening to music, it has no negative side effects, and nowadays it is highly portable. So why not give it a try? Once you see the benefits of music in terms of relaxation, you will realize it is an ally both in preventing disease and in reducing symptoms inherent to any diseases you might already have.

Keep in tune with the mind and the heart will follow. The mind is the bandleader and the heart is the orchestra; it's really your choice how and what you play.

HEART ON

A Poem and a Prayer

In this pit
I am reaching
And my hands seem blurred

And tired
I am tired
Of crying to myself
I miss you
You who lived as me
With my name and spirit
I want you back
And loving.
Seems like it will never
Be the same,
As I am not the same.
What is this place called
Need?
So crowded
So lonely, so full of itself?

As my tired thoughts
     yawn
I receive your
     Energy
To be able to continue
Through
The paradox
Of doing
     And doing without

Heart Song

BETH M., *nurse practitioner and holistic healer, Sarasota, Florida, and Sag Harbor, New York*

I've owned a holistic women's health-care practice for the past twenty-two years. I do a lot of work with hypothyroidism, adrenal fatigue, and heart disease. And I've wondered for a while, What's going on with women and their hearts? My professional opinion is that our modern lifestyle places too much strain and stress on us. We don't take enough care of our health, in the holistic sense of mind, body, and spirit.

But what I want to talk about specifically here is a very common problem among women: broken heart syndrome. A study published in the February 2005 *New England Journal of Medicine* confirmed what I've known for a long time to be true: A tragic or shocking event can produce classic heart attack–like symptoms, such as chest pain, shortness of breath, rapid heartbeat, and fluid in the lungs. Fortunately, recovery from broken heart syndrome is physically much easier than recovery from a real heart attack. But the emotional recovery is an entirely different story. And

I have a story of my own about BHS that I'd like to share.

About four years ago, a wonderful man came into my life—or so I thought. I was fifty-seven years old at the time. He decided that I was his true love and announced that he wanted to spend the rest of his life with me. He was married, but he left his marriage when I said I wouldn't see him unless he was single. We had amazing times together sailing and skiing and sharing life emotionally and physically. Things started to get serious and we were making plans to spend our lives together. I had finally connected to my soul mate, and the future looked very fulfilling. It seemed a miracle that at this point in my life I was going to have some real happiness.

Then it all fell to pieces. One day, I asked if he was seeing anyone besides me. He said he was—many other women, I was soon to discover. And that wasn't all; he also confessed that he was going to strip joints and getting lap dances on a regular basis. This was very upsetting to me because I'd waited a long time to be with someone, and I honestly believed he was the love of my life. I didn't understand how he could do these things.

When he first told me about the other women, I started crying hysterically. I felt betrayed and unsafe. My heart rate rapidly escalated to 173 beats per minute. I went to the cardiologist to have a stress test, and he told me that I had ventricular tachycardia. He said that if I didn't go on meds immediately, I could go into heart failure. I was terrified. The next morning, I went to the drugstore to get my beta-blockers. But I didn't want to take them. I was seeing an expert homeopath and a naturopath at the time, and so I decided this was the type of treatment I preferred. I didn't buy the drugs; I got myself a stuffed panda instead. When I got home, I called my natural-medicine practitioners and was given a homeopathic remedy to calm the heart. I also took some natural hormones to balance the hormones that had gone haywire from the stress response.

After conducting extensive research on my own, I found out that the stress response is a major contributor to heart disease. Yet most practitioners seem to focus on diet, exercise, and laboratory numbers, without discussing the stress hormones and their effect on the heart at all. I realized that I had broken heart syndrome. You see, when you're under stress, your body puts out huge amounts of cortisol and epinephrine. These stress hormones make your heart beat rapidly and create a hormonal imbalance. I knew that the only way to cure myself was to end the relationship. So that's what I did. My "true love" admitted that he was a sex addict and said he was not willing to seek treatment, so I suggested he go back to his wife, who could pretend not to know. And that's what he did.

To me, this story is such a vivid demonstration of the mind-body connection. Look at what an addictive relationship, devastation, and depression can do to your heart! Staying healthy and preventing heart disease is not just about getting proper nutrition and exercise; it's also about managing your stress. This is the whole basis of my practice with women. I'm working with what I myself must learn. But my experience, as awful as it was, has helped me encourage my clients to take a good look at their lives and their relationships. Avoiding illness is not just about taking meds; it's about changing your life. If you don't, you *will* get sick. I had to let go of this relationship in order to save myself. My lover wasn't willing to give up his addiction, and I wasn't willing to give up my heart.

Let me make a cautionary statement here. One of the reasons why women get misdiagnosed when they are suffering from heart attacks is because doctors tell them that they're just having an anxiety attack. If you're having symptoms of heart disease, please don't just dismiss them as being due to broken heart syndrome and stay home. Go to your doctor and get tested. It's entirely possible that you do have heart disease and need professional care. At the same time, I think that when people have heart attacks, doctors should ask, "What's going on in your life, in your relationships?" Because stress hormones are so powerful, they really can change the dynamics. I've seen it with cancer, too. They suppress your immune system. There's always a bigger picture.

My heart problems haven't come back at all since I got over that man. I'm dancing, I'm having a good time, I feel healthy, I look younger, and I feel younger. So remember: I'm not saying you shouldn't have your heart checked out just because you're going through some life trauma—you always should. But keep in mind the critical link that exists between your heart and everything else that's going on in your life. Each exerts a powerful influence over the other.

I'm not down on love these days. Love can break your heart, but it can also heal your heart. Now that I've had this experience with broken heart syndrome, I'm able to help other women heal better. I'm able to look at their physical as well as emotional symptoms with deeper compassion and insight. And in the end, the goal is always healing.

6.

THE WHITE SALE: EVERYTHING MUST GO

If you are irritated by every rub, how will you be polished?

—RUMI

Slowly, like clouds burn off on a gloomy June morning in Malibu, my depressive fog was beginning to see light. Either that or it was becoming an integrated part of the emerging new me. I felt a deep longing to return to some semblance of my old, familiar life. The problem was that as soon as I began to recover from the physical and psychological hardships this trauma had put me through, I was knocked flat on my face by financial hardship. What can stop a person who would never stop before? Take away her health and then her money. I'd been distracting myself, allowing denial to set in, but high noon had arrived in red ink. Quite simply, I was broke.

The Heart Truth

**Bypass surgeries can cost more than
$100,000 if complications arise.**

—*FAST COMPANY*, 2005

Where had all my savings gone? Well, I was three years and change into the healing process. There were so many exceptional expenses: medicines, vitamins and herbs to counter the horrible side effects of the medicines, numerous alternative treatments for body and spirit, and checking in with countless doctors to get their opinions on why this had happened to me. Not to mention all the usual expenses—house, car, food, pet care, insurance, and so on—and the fact that I hadn't earned a penny for some time now.

Heart Song

MARY D., *Kansas City, Kansas*

I used to be a runner. I used to teach aerobics classes at several different levels. But ever since I got heart disease last year at age sixty-three, I can't do that stuff anymore. I don't have much mobility. I cry a lot. And I've completely run out of money.

My heart disease showed up out of the blue. I was in the middle of an advanced aqua-aerobics class when my heart rate shot up to 170 and would not drop. The doctors diagnosed atrial fibrillation and performed two surgeries. I wish I knew what caused it, but I don't. No one has a clue. The cardiologist wants to implant a pacemaker now, but I won't allow it. I feel like it would mean killing a large portion of my heart.

I have really struggled with the lack of a support system. Many of the important men in my life can't or won't deal with my heart disease, which has resulted in my having more emotional and psychological problems. You've got to look for a female support network. (See the appendix, page 199, which offers resources for women with heart disease.)

I've also had a terrible time dealing with health insurance. People with chronic issues frequently can't get health insurance. Or if they did have it, they are dropped. The only thing that saves them is if they can get on a group policy under someone else's name. I have tried some of the "low-cost clinics." But I find that these doctors just want to get you out the door as quickly as possible, so they tend to overprescribe medications. The best doctor who will see me now is sixty-three miles away, and the closest ER that will take me without health insurance is forty minutes away. I guess that's just the way it is.

—————

It's true: Money can't buy you health (or love), but it *can* buy what you need to survive and live on, especially health care in today's world. And I had an entirely different definition of health care than most people. I had an exquisite yoga teacher, Micheline, who studied how heart patients should move after their surgery and helped me reconnect with my body in a respectful and empowering way. I did Pilates and weight training to strengthen my muscles, cardio exercise by walking on the beach with Sage, and chi gung to maintain my balance. I had hands-on energy work and acupuncture, which always gave me a boost. I had Indian hot oil massages. I had my skin rolled, a process whereby the masseuse basically pinches every part of your skin and pulls it away from the bone to keep it vital and supple. My friend John Steele concocted scented oils to help diminish my scars and keep my spirits alive. I worked with a dream interpreter to decipher where my internal process was taking me. I did it all and it did me.

♡ *Since as women we all come with the same parts but different operating instructions, disease and recovery work differently for each one of us.*

Dietwise, I naturally shopped at the farmer's market every week, choosing from the cornucopia of organic foods.

My staples were fruits and veggies, soups, and whole grains, as always, but I had started desiring more protein—fish, chicken, and even a lamb chop or two. I'd been a healthy eater for decades, but now I gave myself a wider berth to explore. Never a chocolate fan before (yes, I know that eliminates me from the Women's Club), I became an avid connoisseur of pure bittersweet chocolate. I introduced soy lattes. And after years and years of not drinking, I also started to enjoy a glass of red wine here and there, as the doctors recommended for my type of heart disease. Slowly, these helped me regain my appetite for life.

The Heart Truth

Red wine (no more than two glasses per night) and dark chocolate (at least 70 percent pure) are pleasant dietary recommendations for most women with heart disease. They both seem to help the body process cholesterol. Enjoy!

—DR. JESSE HANLEY

The standard meds that doctors prescribe for postsurgery heart disease patients were not for me; I had some kind of reaction whenever I took them. There is no such thing as a standard regimen for women with heart disease anyway, just as there is no such thing as a standard hormone treatment that works for every woman. There is a protocol that doctors usually follow, but not everyone fits into those guidelines. I was, as usual, a misfit. So I convinced the doctors to let me try red yeast rice, an all-natural alternative to Lipitor, to reduce my cholesterol. My cholesterol went down sixty points.

In addition, I did chelation treatments. The substance EDTA is injected into your blood via an IV drip for two-plus hours each session. It then binds with heavy metals (such as lead) and the plaque they leave behind, thereby helping your body secrete these unhealthy elements through your urine. Although there's no FDA approval for chelation and the sessions left me shaky at times, I still believe in it because it worked: My angina symptoms began to diminish.

So, yes, all these treatments cost money, sometimes lots of money, and insurance doesn't cover most of the alternative approaches. The realities were pressing in; I had to get back to work. If only I knew what I felt like doing, or was capable of doing, then I could move forward. But I had no clue.

The Heart Truth

The age-adjusted rate of heart disease is 72 percent higher for African-American women than for Caucasian women. African-American women ages fifty-five to sixty-four are twice as likely as Caucasian women to have a heart attack and 35 percent more

likely to suffer from coronary artery disease. This is partly due to the fact that African-American women are more likely to be obese and have diabetes.

—AHA, 2005

Now that death had come knocking and I had no children, I felt more certain than ever that I needed to leave a legacy behind. I wondered what my gifts and passions could conjure up before I left this planet. I'd always believed the greatest gift I had was the way I could inspire people to change. I'd lived my life in nonstop change mode and now, looking back, knew it to be my greatest teacher. I also believed that women can be an amazing catalyst for change. I'd dreamed many times of creating events where women could gather to listen and share their stories. I believe that one woman will tell her own story but that many women will tell the *whole* story. Storytelling is the most powerful tool we have as a culture. I wondered if I might find a way to make this a reality: to bring women together in order to effect change.

Serendipitously, I connected with my old friend Carole, a successful film and TV producer. We had known each other for over twenty years. She shared my vision, and so together we began developing a plan to bring our ideas to fruition. She'd known me in the years when my magic was still available, so working with her was not a reminder of what had just happened; rather, it was a confirmation of the Pamela who could do anything. And that was the Pamela I needed again now.

♡ *The soul, if given the chance, will dance you right to the end.*

Heart Song

CAROLE ISENBERG, *Pamela's close friend,*
New York, New York

It was the summer of 1981 when I first met Pamela. I was living in Los Angeles and Pamela, who lived in New York, was visiting one of my close friends. She was a sprite with short dark hair, luminous brown-cherry eyes, a wide, disarming, bucktoothed smile, and big energy. Pamela was designing unique jewelry in those days. But she was always looking at the alchemical nature of life, seeking the opportunity to express herself in as many creative mediums as possible. We clicked right away—the way people do when you speak the same language. My mother was dying of breast cancer and there was a lot of shame attached to the disease at the time, but Pamela didn't mind talking about it.

As we lived our busy lives on separate coasts, we kept in touch. But our contact became more and more sporadic, and for several years we lost touch completely. And then one day, there was Pamela on the phone, her familiar husky voice telling me she was moving to L.A. "I have decided to change my life," she said. "How fantastic!" I replied. She promised to call once she was settled.

Well, I didn't hear from her for six months, and when she did call, she had quite a story to tell. Not possible, I thought, not possible that Pamela had triple bypass surgery. We made plans for dinner. I remember pulling up to her house in Malibu. She was tan and sitting on the front step, waiting for me. I got out of the car and walked over to her and we hugged. Then we pulled back and took a good look at each other. Pamela was more woman and less sprite. She was wearing a bright green V-necked T-shirt that showed off the thin line of her scar. It was her own beauty mark.

As we rekindled our friendship, I saw that Pamela's heart event had had a profound effect on her life. The Pamela I'd met in the eighties wanted to be everywhere and do everything. Not so this woman. There was fragility to her energy now. She was careful about how much she put out and how many people were around her at a time. I found her more thoughtful, introspective, compassionate, and humble.

Having a close friend with heart disease has been an education for me. I did not realize that heart disease was the number-one killer of women. I did not know that the signs of a woman having a heart attack are different from those of a man. I take stress tests regularly now and I'm very aware of any new research being done. Because of Pamela, I truly understand what it means to live a heart-healthy life.

Heart disease isn't a condition that is cured. You don't just go on as you did before. Heart disease is a condition that you live with forever. It is, as Pamela says, "a new normal." But this isn't necessarily a bad thing. I feel that Pamela, as a survivor, has greater appreciation for the simple fact that she is alive—and so do I.

After five years in L.A., I felt like I was getting sick of the light, the sun, the salsa, and the smoothie generation. Maybe being in L.A. was just too reminiscent of everything, too much cell memory here of recovering from my heart surgery. I needed to cleanse my palate.

♡ *Our hearts have everything to do with what our minds imagine they conceived.*

Around that time, Carole and I began working on a project together with Revlon and Almay called "Making Up," a series of vignettes we performed on how women transform themselves from the inside out, from their makeup to their emotions. It was so much fun. We were smitten with the idea of performance as a way to spread information. Spending time in NYC for the presentation, I realized how much I missed my family and how much I missed the Pamela I was when I lived there, before all this had happened. I craved the real bagels as well as the clamor, smells, and creatures of Manhattan. Dorothy had it right: There's no place like home. So Habebe and I drove across the country and I felt like a kid again, with dreams in my pocket and hope in my heart.

The Heart Truth

Several mild risks, such as slight elevations in blood pressure and cholesterol levels due to stress, can pose more of a threat to women's heart health than one major risk, such as having diabetes or smoking.
—JOHNS HOPKINS UNIVERSITY SCHOOL OF MEDICINE, 2005

Well, it turns out my memory of New York City was much better than the reality of what it—or I—had become. As soon as I returned, I started to question my decision. No, you never really can go home again; this was certainly true for me. The grass was indeed greener on the other coast. Immediately I longed for the softness of L.A., the palm trees, the humidity-free sunshine, the calming sound of waves. I remembered how slowly I moved there, so contrary to my constant rush down the streets of Manhattan. Here, my heart quickened at the noise, the commotion, and the smells of garbage in the August heat. In spite of the pain I'd suffered there, the West Coast had provided me with healing space, room to breathe and see my life without the drive and clutter that NYC had always embodied in me. I felt like I was neither here nor there, sushi nor pastrami.

Being in Manhattan immediately revved me up to a pace that I knew I could not sustain. I thought that by returning home I'd be able to reconnect with the places inside myself where I was powerful, successful, and effective. But that was magical thinking—and I was no longer a magician.

I have met many women who think the way to the heart is to chart its course rationally, eat the right food, reduce stress, and exercise. While these are all important parts of the prescription for a healthy life, they are by no means the only ones. For me, if the obvious cause of my heart disease was my family history, the secret cause was the way I metabolized stress hormones. I cooked stress up as drama and gobbled it down like a gourmand devouring a loaf of hot, crusty bread. Then I'd let it stew inside me for days, even weeks, on end, like a spicy pasta sauce, and either flambé it or store it away. When I stowed stress, guess where it landed? Smack-dab in the middle of my heart. So here I was again, letting NYC do what it does best: stress me out. I feared and felt another episode coming on, as most heart patients do, and I was right.

♡ *Nature remains constant in renewing its flaws.*

HEALING THE HEART

Hormones, Menopause, and Heart Disease

By Erika Schwartz, M.D., author of *Natural Energy, The Hormone Solution, The 30-Day Natural Hormone Plan,* and *Dr. Erika's Hormone Solution for Your Daughter*

I'd like to explore the connection between hormones and heart disease. Postmenopausal women are more likely to get heart disease because estrogen and progesterone, which become depleted with the onset of menopause, no longer protect their hearts. As the levels of these hormones drop, the incidence of heart disease in women skyrockets and their statistics catch up with those for men. If a woman also smokes, is under constant stress, and does not take care of herself, her risk for heart disease becomes even higher with age than a man's.

Unfortunately, it can be difficult for a doctor to tell

the difference between heart disease and menopause in women because the symptoms can be so similar: exhaustion, general fatigue, foggy thinking, nausea, palpitations, anxiety attacks, night sweats, frequent urination, mood swings, and bloating. However, with heart disease, these symptoms rapidly worsen within a period of hours to minutes, whereas with menopause, they often fluctuate and are usually self-limited.

Doctors *must* conduct routine baseline cardiac evaluations, stress testing, and overall evaluations of lifestyle for *all* menopausal women in order to rule out the presence of heart disease. If your doctor doesn't do this for you at your next physical exam, be sure to ask him or her to do it.

Symptoms of menopause can be treated with bioidentical hormones, proper supplements, a hormone-friendly diet, exercise, and stress-management programs. All of these treatments will also help decrease the severity of heart problems if already present. Bioidentical hormones are prescription hormones that are molecularly identical to the hormones our bodies make naturally and in balance when we are young. They are less likely than synthetic hormones to produce adverse side effects (as discovered in the large-scale Women's Health Initiative study). The most commonly used bioidentical hormones are estradiol, micronized progesterone, and micronized testosterone. Hormone-friendly diets are high in lean protein, vegetables, and fruits and low in hormone busters, such as foods containing trans-fatty acids, animal fats, processed carbs, and starches, as well as coffee, soda, and alcohol. Physical activity and stress management are also crucial ingredients in maintaining a hormonally balanced lifestyle, which translates into a healthy heart at any age or stage of life.

My advice to women of all ages is this: Live in your body; be aware of the way it functions and the messages it continuously sends to you. Don't ignore these signs. Also, do not be intimidated into becoming a victim of either conventional or alternative medical treatments. Listen to all your options and make your own choices. Start by taking control of your lifestyle, diet, sleep, exercise, and, above all, attitude. Ask questions about the pills and supplements you are taking. Do you really need them all?

Don't waste your time worrying and asking, "Why me?" Why *not* you? Your genetics, environment, or just your life in general have brought you here. Wasting precious energy wondering why won't improve your health today or help you live a better tomorrow. Take responsibility for making your life healthier and longer. Life is short and we never know when it will end. You may be afflicted with heart disease, but that doesn't mean you know for sure that heart disease will kill you. You may walk out the door and get run over by a car first, or you may live on as a survivor of heart disease for many years to come by taking good care of yourself and keeping your hormones in balance. My thirty years of experience have shown that the better your attitude, the more likely you are to survive longer and continue to enjoy a successful, healthy life.

HEART ON

Healing Ritual

Whenever my finances get the better of me and I get depressed about it, I do this ritual: I write a check to myself for the amount of money that I need. In the memo part of the check, I put where the funds are coming from and why—for example, "Cure for heart disease." Then I mail it to myself. When I receive it and open it, I always feel better. Often, unexpected loans or income from spontaneous sources find their way to me at the very same time.

I know it may seem a little out there, but at this point, what more do you have to lose? Try it. Just pick the number that makes you feel more empowered in your life, write it down on the dotted line, sign, and allow the miracle and energy of your intention to see you through.

Heart Song

LEESANN S., *Palm Desert, California*

My story is a little different. I don't have heart disease, per se. Rather, I was born with three holes in my heart. Until I had heart surgery at the age of ten, I would literally turn blue whenever I exerted myself too much. My early life unfolded under all kinds of restrictions. I wasn't allowed to run, play, or laugh like other children, for fear that it would over-burden my heart. I wasn't even supposed to cry! When something bad happened that upset me, my grand-mother would hold me throughout the night to make sure that I didn't break down and start sobbing. Sometimes I'd fall asleep on one shoulder and my mother would fall asleep on the other, and we'd spend the whole night that way, until we had to get up for work and school. It gave me a very strong sense of family. I feel so blessed for all the sacrifices my mom and grandparents made for me.

I'd always wanted to dance. When I was four, one of the girls at our church gave me a pair of toe shoes. I put them on, walked over to my mom, who was do-ing the laundry, and said, "I'm going to be a dancer when I grow up!" My mom stopped putting the clothes in the washing machine and looked at me. "That's never going to happen," she said. But I just looked right back at her and said, "Yes, I *am* going to be a dancer." She said, "You have a special heart. But we're going to try to fix it. We're going to meet some doctors and you're going to have an operation. But that can't happen until you're older."

When I reached age ten, the doctors were finally ready to perform the surgery. They didn't want to wait too long because they didn't think I'd live past twelve, but they also couldn't do it too soon because they knew it would be a real shock to my system. They were right. It was a difficult road to recovery. My lungs collapsed and I got pneumonia, so they had to redo the surgery. I remember the doctor saying the very next day, "We have to do a tracheotomy." They had me packed in ice. It was intense.

Well, I don't know where it came from, but the will to live was so strong in me. I was ferocious. My defiance saved me. I was able to direct it in a very constructive manner toward recovering from my open-heart surgery. I kept saying to myself, I'm going to live, and I'm going to do what I feel called to do. I'm going to live *my* way.

As soon as I was well, I discovered, to my sheer delight, that my problems were solved. My energy levels increased exponentially. No more restrictions! I was free to run, laugh, play, and cry. And I became a dancer for life. I started taking tap lessons, baton lessons. I'd say to my girlfriends, "Let's do that dance from *Mary Poppins*!" Then we would, and I'd think, Oh my gosh, I can really do this now! To a child who couldn't do any of this before, it was a really big deal. I even majored in dance at college.

When I was in my mid-twenties, I came to a place of peace inside myself. I realized that my heart was strong. It didn't have to do with the physical strength; it was the strength of having something greater, the strength of my heart being not just me. Our hearts are connected to the planet, the planet is our mother, and the planet has a rhythm. The essence of nurturing is universal. The strength of the heart doesn't come from the one; it comes from the many. Those may sound like clichés, but they're so true for me.

Now I'm fifty. My lungs still aren't real strong. I can't run fast, and I never learned to swim. But I can dance. When you're dancing, it's not just you. There's God, there's the music, and there's what you're giving back to whoever is watching. You're being carried. To this day, I consider myself a very heart-oriented person, and I have dedicated myself to helping others. Interesting how a calling can be born of what's missing sometimes, isn't it?

I was told when I was ten that I'd never be able to have children. But in college, I had a bunch of tests done, and they told me that I would. What a blessing it was to hear that news! My son, Evin, was born with a heart condition as well, though not as serious as mine. He has pulmonary stenosis, which means that the artery going into his left lung is slightly narrower than the one going into his right. He's going to have a stent put in, but it should all work out just fine. Thankfully, modern medicine is way beyond where it was when I was little. My husband, Jacob, and I tell him that he has a very special "lion's heart," because his heartbeat is so loud that it sounds like a lion's roar!

If you'd like my advice for how to deal with your heart issues, here it is:

1. Always ask for help from the "unseen worlds."
2. Find what you love doing, and do lots of it.
3. Find a doctor or specialist whom you really trust.

7.

WHERE IT STOPS,
NOBODY KNOWS

Let life happen to you. Believe me: life is in the right, always.
—RAINER MARIA RILKE

It's Thursday, December 18, 2003, and Christmas is everywhere. Even with the blustering cold wind, shoppers swarm the city, fearlessly navigating the thick applesauce slush that covers the streets. Store windows overflowing with fancy and fattening foods flirt with people's preholiday resolutions. Colorful cashmere temptations along Madison Ave cry out to my inner addict. Horns honk and traffic crawls. In other words, it's business as usual in NYC.

On this otherwise-normal day, I set off to negotiate my way through the sludge to meet my new cardiologist, Dr. Jane Farhi. Much as I'd like to deny it, I've been having chest pains again. So here I am, an hour and counting, waiting for my appointment, when all I really want to do is bolt and window-shop while sipping a frothy cappuccino. Some things never change.

♡ *Heart disease is forever.*

Dr. Farhi is charming, smart, and attentive. I can tell within two minutes that we're a good fit. We speak about my old and new symptoms, and I am struck by something she says after reviewing my chart. "You have advanced arteriosclerosis." By this, she doesn't mean that I belong in a gifted or master's-level class, but, rather, that, having had my first heart event at age forty-seven, it's likely my heart disease will return again and again. I also take it to mean I'm looking at twenty more years of life at best.

Next, we proceed to the treadmill for a stress test. Two minutes, five minutes, and I'm still feeling all right. But at eight minutes, I start to feel distressed. Dr. Farhi suddenly gets pale and looks up from the machines. "We need to get you to the hospital immediately," she says.

"No way, no way," I reply, face flushing. This can't be happening again.

"You have the signs of an impending heart attack."

"Right now?" I counter.

"Yes, right now," she repeats as she gets paler and I get more agitated.

"You mean right this minute right now, or it's coming? The anticipation is the hardest part."

"It's sort of like hearing a tornado approaching without being able to see it. You notice the colors change and the air takes on a claustrophobic demeanor. If you are not having a heart attack now, you are on the brink and it could happen any second," she explains.

"How does a heart attack get close?" I ask.

She shows me the graph. There is a big blip, but there are so many blips. I start to break down. "How can we be sure? I cannot do this again, I just can't. I won't make it."

I burst out crying. Dr. Farhi tries to comfort me, and her own eyes fill with tears. She says, "I have no choice; you have no choice. We both know the truth. You are in danger of a heart attack now, and I won't let you go home. You must go directly to the emergency room. This can't wait." Does she think it's the first time I've heard this line? I know the routine. What I want to know is this: Who screwed up and put Groundhog Day in the middle of December?

What is the difference between heartache and heart disease? Answer: the hospital. It isn't the emergency room that I fear, but the room beyond it, the operating room. I have had just about all that I can take. If a cat has nine lives, how many does the human heart have? And how much more can I take? That seems to be the question of my lifetime.

The Heart Truth

**Thirty-five percent of female, versus 18 percent
of male, heart attack survivors will have
another heart attack within six years.**

—WOMENHEART, 2005

I ask to forgo the ambulance. I've done that before and discovered that it's not as much fun as it looks. So I walk slowly out the door, feeling so disappointed in myself, as if I've had everything to do with this, and frightened that it is another ending. A heart attack for Christmas, the gift that keeps on giving. I climb into a taxi. "Lenox Hill emergency room, please."

Heart Song

JUNE B., *Rockville, Maryland*

I had an aortic-valve replacement and a single bypass in May of 2004, when I was sixty-seven. My heart disease was partially congenital, because I was born with a bicuspid rather than a tricuspid valve. I also knew that heart disease was in my family. My father died of heart failure at seventy-six. Since I have a medical background (I'm a retired microbiologist with a Ph.D.), I was aware that heart disease was something that would probably happen to me.

Prior to my surgery, I was asymptomatic and athletic, but also a smoker and overweight. In 1996, my gynecologist noted my high blood pressure and sent me to a cardiologist. We controlled the high blood pressure with meds and a low-salt diet for about three years. In the following two years, I had several echocardiograms and thallium stress tests, which revealed that my heart problems were getting worse. An angiogram in February 2004 told the full story: I was to prepare myself for an aortic-valve replacement—the sooner the better.

I consider myself very lucky. I had plenty of time to make preparations and interview a number of doctors to find the most experienced one available. I also got to choose between a mechanical and tissue valve, weighing the pros and cons of each type. The mechanical valve meant taking Coumadin, an anticoagulant, for the rest of my life, but the tissue valve could wear out in ten years. My sister-in-law had had to get her tissue valve replaced after eight years, when she was seventy-nine. Normally, they do not replace valves at that age, but she was in quite good health, so she lucked out. I opted for the mechanical valve and Coumadin, even though taking it means that you constantly have to monitor diet and INR values (the "thinness" or "thickness" of your blood), you bruise easily, and you cannot engage in risky physical activities.

I went into surgery with a very positive attitude. I was joking around with the doctors and nurses. You're not supposed to wear any makeup or jewelry, but I had a pedicure just before the procedure. Later, the hospital staff remembered me, saying, "Oh, you're the lady with the pretty toes!" My surgery went well and I was discharged after just four days.

After the surgery, my cardiologist proposed a course at a cardiac rehab center. I'd always been an active person, a tap dancer and tennis player, but I'd slowed down a bit. Now I'm an avid exerciser at the rehab center. Most women my age or older don't continue with their rehab program. I figure maybe they're embarrassed to sweat. But I embrace it. I'm proud that I can now maintain a steady heart rate for a vigorous forty- to fifty-minute workout three days a week. I've also stopped smoking, lost fifteen pounds, and am enjoying eating a healthy low-salt diet. A year after my surgery, at the age of sixty-eight, I feel wonderful and my doctors says my heart is in great shape!

My attitude about life is that you wait out the low points and relish the high points, knowing that neither will continue forever. So when the doctors told me I had to change my lifestyle because of my heart disease, I changed. I said to myself, I have to do this. I have to take care of myself. I hope you'll do the same.

The Heart Truth

About half the time, bypass grafts clog up within a few years, angioplasties within a few months.

—AHA, 2005

Needless to say, I survived the heart episode in NYC. And now on my record, it shows I did have a small heart attack. The doctors put a medicated stent inside the section of artery that was clogged. They said this stent would defy plaque buildup and allow the artery to stay open longer than the nonmedicated type would. It was twenty-four hours of anguish for me, yet I got to check out of the hospital the very next day. Yes, apparently the operation is as simple and routine as taking out tonsils. At least that's what they tell you. Nothing can make me believe it, no matter how fast or how well the procedure is performed. I was exhausted for weeks afterward.

♡ *For cancer survivors, the constant question is, "Will it come back?" For heart disease survivors, the question is, "Is it still open?"*

I started to sink back into depression. Remember that the heart and depression are sisters; they know when the other is in trouble. The problem was that I'd spent the last five years denying that I really had heart disease. I had written off the bypass as a fluke. It had seemed the only way to move forward in my life. But now, with this petit heart attack and stent procedure, I couldn't lie to myself any longer. The walls of my denial came tumbling down. Humpty-Dumpty was in pieces again.

But a few weeks later, I discovered that underneath all the panic, pain, depression, and frustration, there was a real Chanukah gift waiting for me at, of all places, the waiting room in the doctor's office. What a metaphor. During a follow-up visit to Dr. Farhi, I met a woman who told me about her *five* stent procedures. She said, "What choice do I have? I've learned how to *live with heart disease and be positive about it.*" I felt as though this was the long-awaited message that needed to be delivered to me, that needed to be part of my life now. And so I received it that way.

Hearing the words "learned how to live with heart disease" come out of the mouth of another heart patient rather than from a doctor authenticated my experience. It didn't erase my depression, but it added color, like a kaleidoscope, to my ever-changing emotions. Somehow, I could finally accept that I was a heart survivor and feel okay about it. I knew that I was a strong, capable individual carrying the burden of heart disease along with eight million other women I'd never even met. I felt a surge of energy from the realization in a way I hadn't since all this had begun.

♡ *Allow enough room in the agony of recovery for the ecstasy of being well.*

In that instant, I knew what I needed to do. I was going to write my story, to get it off my own chest finally. And I was going to get the stories off the chests of many other women who were carrying their burdens, suffering from them, and recycling them into multiple events for themselves. We are our own stories until we write them or speak them, and then we become part of the collective consciousness that holds those stories. Once that happens, we no longer feel isolated. I needed to spread the message about heart disease in women. I needed to take on the marketing job no one else wanted: selling heart disease to women to help them save their own lives. I wasn't sure I knew how to do it, but regardless, I was certainly going to give it a try.

The Heart Truth

One study showed that women are 40 percent less likely than men to be diagnosed as suffering from a heart attack.

—*SENIOR JOURNAL,* 2005

But first I realized that I would really, finally, have to learn how to deal with my own stress. I was still an over-the-top responder to events in my life. I would have made a great fireman, but as a heart patient, maintaining this instant alert system was not in my best interest. Why could I not give each event a minute to soak in before reacting to it? What did I have to lose? And so at long last, I taught myself all the things I'd taught *other* people for decades: how to center myself, how to breathe, how to let go of the anxiety. Calm down, I would tell myself. Is all this worrying worth what it's robbing from you? Do you want to give yourself another heart event? That last question usually stopped me in my tracks.

♡ *Interview your cardiologist—in advance of any procedures, if possible—to make sure that there is an open-door policy, one inclusive of your anxiety. Pick a cardiologist who realizes that anxiety and depression are inevitable partners with heart disease. Otherwise, you might find yourself being medicated for anxiety while your actual heart symptoms fall by the wayside.*

In addition, I discovered a fabulous support network. I Googled "women and heart disease" and found an advocacy group called WomenHeart. It is a nonprofit organization that works solely on behalf of women with heart disease. The director, Nancy Loving, immediately connected me to a lunch group of female heart survivors in NYC. It was love at first bite. These women were embracing, funny, informative, inclusive, and nourishing.

The Heart Truth

Social isolation and heart disease are interwined.
Don't live your life in emotional exile.
Find a support network.
—WOMENHEART, 2005

The next year, I received a scholarship from Women-Heart to go to the Mayo Clinic for five days, along with fifty other women from across the country, to learn about all aspects of heart disease. The purpose of the course was to teach us how to communicate through our communities and the media the news about this unbelievable epidemic facing modern American women. We studied every topic from diet to depression, from procedures to poetry. Doctors shared results from the most impressive and current research studies. Other patients weighed in with their opinions. We laughed, we cried, and, most of all, we didn't deny what this disease feels like. It was an incredibly healing event, and it gave me so many women to keep up the dialogue with about heart disease.

Heart Song

———

FAITH T., *Orange City, Florida*

I'm forty-eight years old now, but I started having problems with my heart when I was about twenty-one. The problem was that at age sixteen I was diagnosed with hypothyroidism (meaning my thyroid wasn't active enough), and so my doctor put me on thyroid-replacement medication. Then I moved from Florida to Chicago, so it was five months before I got to a doctor for a checkup. During those five months, I lost about fifty pounds, had no energy, and was very sick. It hurt to swallow, it hurt to eat. The doctor discovered three goiters growing around my esophagus because my thyroid had become overactive. I underwent surgery to have the goiters removed.

At the same time, I started having a lot of chest pain and heart palpitations. I went to see a cardiologist. He told me that during this period of thyroid hyperactivity (due to the same drugs that had caused the goiters), a valve in my heart had been damaged. He put me on meds; I don't remember what. I took them because I was young and stupid and didn't understand anything.

Two years later, I moved back to Florida. I kept

going to cardiologists because I was experiencing the sensation of someone grabbing my heart, squeezing it for thirty seconds, and then letting it go. That would happen a few times in a row. At first, it happened every few months, but over the years it progressed to the point where it was happening daily. I went to a bunch of different doctors, and they tried all kinds of meds, but nothing helped. All they could tell me was that my tests looked normal and they couldn't explain what was going on with my heart.

When I first went to the doctor I have now, he asked me about my family history. When he realized that my father had suffered three heart attacks by the age of sixty-five, he said genetics had probably contributed to my heart problems, along with the drugs I'd been inappropriately treated with in my youth. He did a cardiac catheterization and prescribed some new meds, which have helped. It's the closest any doctor has come yet to fixing things with my heart.

Heart disease has definitely affected my life. For one thing, I get tired out extremely easily. Trying to hold down a full-time job is very difficult. Just walking across the office and back, I get so winded that I have to sit down for a few minutes to rest. I'm also very aware of my own mortality.

Luckily, I was able to have children, which was a great surprise. My husband and I had tried for four years to have a child, and then one day it just happened. It was scary because it was only five months after the goiter surgery and we had planned to wait at least a year, but our son is a great kid, as is our daughter. I have a four-year-old grandson now. Because of him, I'm careful to monitor what I eat, exercise, and keep the extra weight off. I want to be around to watch him grow up.

Today is July 28, 2005, my fifty-fourth birthday, and I finally can say that I understand the gifts that heart disease has bestowed on me. Heart disease has become the greatest teacher in my life. My heart was always the biggest and strongest part of me, though it proved to be also the most vulnerable. Today, those two facts are integrated, not separated. And for the most part, I am reenchanted with life, though of course I still have "heart off" days. In spite of the pain, I would not trade a day of all the growth. They were my journey back to myself.

So now I have written my memoir and my friend Carol and I are putting on the Broadway benefit *Events of the Heart*. Think of it as *The Angina Monologues*. I eat what I love, I taste experiences with the right balance of caution and abandon, and I am guided by the fact that each and every moment is an opportunity to be in grace. I realize more than ever how to invite God into my life continually, knowing that everything is uncertainty but faith.

All I ever really wanted to do in all my many careers was to spread *heart*. Heart disease has given me the chance to do just that. Here the opportunity was all along, ticking inside me, right at the center of my being.

♡ *You never know where the YES will turn up amid the ocean of nos.*

Since talking is one of the things women do best, let's use our voices—our deep, passionate voices—to break the silence, crack the code, and come into conversation about why heart disease is claiming the lives of so many American women. We deserve more thorough medical research, better equipment, proper diagnosis, and improved treatment—and we are demanding it. Do you realize how powerful we really are? Behind the picket fences and wisteria hedges, in houses, and in offices, women take everything to heart and are at the heart of everything. Did you know that we're responsible for 80 percent of all consumer purchases and 60 percent of the wealth? We could change heart disease policies in this country with a one-day shopping boycott! That would certainly get some attention.

Let's do it. Let's make heart disease our juiciest gossip, our best-selling cover story, our hottest new tip. Let's take it on and not let go until we can walk all together, openhearted. Yes, it's true, we women truly have always been the real heart-on for each other.

The Heart Truth

Use the "alphabet approach" to remember your heart-healthy habits: Take aspirin daily if you're over sixty, keep your blood pressure and cholesterol levels down, don't smoke cigarettes, practice good dietary habits, and exercise regularly.

—JOHNS HOPKINS UNIVERSITY SCHOOL OF MEDICINE, 2005

Changing Your Life

Two years after undergoing coronary artery bypass surgery, 90 percent of people have not changed their lifestyles. Dr. Dean Ornish, however, seems to have come up with a method that works. In 1993, he ran a study (paid for by Mutual of Omaha) in which 333 patients with severely clogged arteries attended twice-weekly group support sessions led by a psychologist, got help quitting smoking, and took instruction in meditation, relaxation, yoga, and aerobic exercise. The program lasted just one year, but after three years, 77 percent of the patients had stuck with their lifestyle changes and had avoided further bypass or angioplasty surgeries. It also saved Mutual of Omaha around $300,000 per patient. Why did it work?

- Dr. Dean Ornish's program avoided using fear of death as a motivator, unlike other programs; rather, it concentrated on promises of a better life. He offered patients an inspired vision of "the joy of living." They talked about such pleasures as what it would be like to feel better, live longer, enjoy walking more, and make love again. "Joy is a more powerful motivator than fear," says Dr. Ornish.

- Appealing to emotions works better than presenting people with a bunch of facts.

—FAST COMPANY, 2005

HEALING THE HEART

Nutrition for Heart Disease

BY SALLY KRAVICH, holistic nutritionist, author of *Vibrant Living: Creating Radiant Health and Longevity*

I've studied health and longevity modalities from around the world: the Amazon, the Middle East, Eastern Europe, Fiji, India, and here in the United States. In my bicoastal practice, I've worked with women for over twenty-five years to improve and integrate the health of body, mind, and soul. Usually, I meet with these women in person to find out their goals and put them on a program of stress management, exercise, food, and nutrients for optimum well-being. Here I'm going to present you with a few general rules that apply to most women with heart disease. However, please consult a physician before implementing any major lifestyle changes.

FOOD

The food that you eat must have the ability to be broken down, absorbed, and eliminated by your body. Here are a few rules to live by, which I call nonnegotiable.

- Get rid of all man-made products. Avoid all fake sugars, fake sweeteners, fake creamers, fake ice cream, and margarine. These products don't have the enzymes contained in real foods, they are insoluble fats, and so our bodies can't break them down. As a result, these fats tend to clump up and form cysts, contributing to illnesses like heart disease, tumors, and cancer.

- Eat plenty of fresh fruits and vegetables. I recommend consuming at least six to eight servings of veggies and two to three servings of fruit per day. Veggies are the repairers. They build new cells and provide nutrients to ensure healing. Fruits are cleansers. One word of caution: People on heart disease medications (e.g., Coumadin, which is a blood thinner) sometimes are told not to consume a lot of dark, leafy greens, such as spinach, dandelion greens, and kale, because these are blood thickeners. However, these veggies are a great source of nutrients, some of the best. So I recommend counteracting the blood-thickening effect by upping your intake of olive oil, fish oil, and sesame seed, which are natural blood thinners. Please be sure to talk to your doctor about this.

- Consume good bacteria. Your body needs healthy bacteria to help you digest your food and absorb all its nutrients. I recommend that my clients consume these bacteria daily. They are found naturally in yogurt. If you're vegan or lactose-intolerant, you can take an acidophilus supplement.

- Eat whole grains. Avoid all products made from white flour, such as white bread and regular pasta, but even keep your consumption of whole wheat low. Try to eat more brown rice, quinoa, millet, rye, and cornmeal instead.

- Consume foods to get your circulatory system moving. Specifically, try to add more cayenne pepper, garlic, and parsley to your diet to help naturally reduce your blood pressure.

- Avoid processed sugar and caffeine. Women these days are generally so stressed that we burn out our adrenal glands, which is terrible for our health. It throws our hormones out of balance and makes us feel exhausted all the time. The usual response to being tired is to consume caffeine and sugar, but the more you do, the worse it gets. You get a temporary rush, but then you come crashing down harder than ever. I advise that you avoid processed sugar and caffeine as much as possible, although it's okay to drink a cup or two of green tea each day.

SUPPLEMENTS

You can't get all the nutrients you need from our over-farmed, overdepleted soil and foods that have been picked, processed, and shipped too often and too soon. So I recommend that you supplement your diet with the following substances.

- Vitamin B complex. These are the antistress vitamins. They nourish the nervous system, help us manage stress and anxiety, and balance our hormones. They're like the electrical wiring in our bodies. Take at least one hundred milligrams per day of vitamin B complex. You may also want to add a little extra B_{12} in order to help your body turn the greens you consume into usable iron, and a folic acid supplement, which promotes heart health. B_6 acts as a natural diuretic, so try to avoid taking it if you're on medications that are diuretics. You should take these vitamins during the day.

- Fatty acids (omega-3, -6, and -9). If B vitamins are the body's electrical wiring, then fatty acids are the insulation tape. The best kind of fatty acid for the heart is fish oil, with flaxseed oil as a second choice. I recommend trying to get your fish oil from wild-caught fresh fish, or frozen if you must. I advise against canned fish because these tend to absorb aluminum from the can. However, you can also take fish- and flaxseed-oil supplements if you don't want to eat fish. It's best to take these at night because they tend to cause burping. Freezing them first and taking them with food will also help alleviate this unpleasant side effect.

- Calcium. Calcium is the grounding cord for your nervous system. It's an emotional and structural support, and it's very important for the heart muscle. Magnesium works well with calcium to help relieve stress, so you can also take a calcium-magnesium supplement. Take these pills at bedtime to help promote good sleep.

- CoQ10. This enzyme helps keep your circulatory system in excellent working order. Take fifty to two hundred milligrams per day, depending on your state of health. Please consult with a health-care specialist to determine how much is right for you.

- Natural substances to reduce cholesterol. Most women with heart disease have high cholesterol levels. To bring your cholesterol levels down naturally, consume plenty of dark, leafy greens and grapefruit, but also try these herbal preparations: Chinese red yeast rice extract and guggal lipids (used in Ayurvedic medicine).

Stress Management

In addition to eating right and consuming the proper supplements, it's crucial to your overall health and wellness that you take care of your body by moving and breathing. I'm a big fan of yoga, which accomplishes both at the same time, and helps reduce stress. Some people enjoy doing cardio exercise as well, which is great. You should exercise at least thirty minutes most days of the week. I also consider massage and deep body work a necessity, not a luxury.

Heart On

Top Heart-ONs and Heart-OFFs

A heart-on is an act of conscious care, a way to feed the soul. The heart thrives on heart-ons; it is the manna from which the heart takes nourishment. Heart attacks or heart-offs are outcries from your heart that your body and soul are in desperate need of attention.

Here are the heart-ons that I live by now, my personal commandments:

1. Putting myself first by saying no to that which doesn't serve me, and giving myself what it is I

really need. (This is the hardest one for women, by the way.)

2. Getting out of my head and learning to find the answers from my heart.

3. Taking time for pleasure, passion, and creativity so that I can be versed in the language of my heart's desires.

4. Taking notice of who I am and what I have, and being aware of and grateful for it all.

5. Expressing love for someone and something every day.

6. Allowing myself and others to be as they are, without judging, blaming, or fixing.

7. Accepting the journey as *right,* just the way it is.

8. Eating with love, as though food were the greatest healer.

9. Moving my body—dancing, walking, stretching, swimming, making love—so that my heart can breathe life in.

10. Listening to and making music that moves my soul.

11. Getting things off my chest; finding ways to express what I feel without reacting to them.

12. Finding peace in moments of chaos, knowing it's usually right there in the middle of the muddle.

13. Allowing balance to be my teacher.

And here are my top heart-offs, the things I try most to avoid:

1. Overdoing, overbeing, overeating, overdrinking, or otherwise abusing myself.
2. Not doing, being, eating, drinking, wearing, or saying what I want.
3. Being in places or with people that don't make me feel alive.
4. Being in toxic relationships with people who cannot meet me in a heartfelt dialogue or who deliver too much drama.
5. Noise, both the kind inside my head and outside it.
6. Traveling down the dark Road of Regrets. Should haves and could haves are lethal, leading to both anger and depression.
7. Being told what is best for me unless I really believe it.
8. Shutting down what I know to be true.
9. Feeling that life has no more surprises in store for me.
10. Placing importance on others' opinions.
11. Going too fast for too long.

Heart Song

Dawn E., *San Jose, California*

It started when I was just twenty-eight years old. It was very much a shock. In May of 2001 my family and I were in Coalinga at a restaurant for a family re-union. I'd just been served my dinner and a margarita. I had just taken my first sip of my cocktail when I started feeling really hot. I pulled my fiancé aside and told him, "I don't feel so good. I think I need to go outside." Because I smoked at the time he thought I wanted to go outside to have a cigarette. "What is it? Please don't tell me you want to have a smoke right now? We just got our food!" he said as he walked me toward the door. By the time we got outside, I had intense pain in my chest and both arms. I felt like I couldn't breathe. I was nauseous and could barely walk. He sat me down in his truck and said, "What's wrong?" "I have to go to the hospital now," I gasped.

Coming from a big city like San Jose, Coalinga felt like the middle of nowhere. The hospital was small and had very few patients; in fact, the lights were dimmed to conserve energy, and there was no one else in the emergency room. I told the doctor that I had tremendous chest pain. He told me, "You're probably having muscle spasms in your chest." They gave me a big shot of muscle relaxants, which helped with the pain. Then they performed an EKG, which came back normal. They were about to send me home when my blood work came back showing that I had sustained heart damage. They wanted to run more tests but weren't equipped to do them at their facility, so I was transported by ambulance to a bigger hospital in Fresno about forty-five minutes away. Once I got there, the doctors kept asking me questions because they couldn't figure out what was going on. Their number one question was, "Are you on drugs?" I kept saying no, because I wasn't and I was confused as to why they kept asking me this question. I had no idea what was going on. They weren't telling me anything. I was also frazzled and very hungry. I'd gone into the hospital at 7:00 P.M. At 10:00 the next morning, they decided to check me in and run further tests.

At 11:00 they finally brought me a sandwich. I was about to take a bite when the doctor came in and said, "Don't eat that! You've had a heart attack." They told me that I would need to have an angiogram, a fairly risky procedure that could cause heart attack, stroke, or even death. I was in total shock. I thought they were going to tell me I'd had a panic attack or heat stroke, as it had been a very hot day. Never did *heart attack* cross my mind. I have no family history of heart disease, no high blood pressure, I'm young, and I wasn't overweight. My cholesterol was on the high end of normal but not yet considered a risk. I just couldn't believe it.

The doctors did the angiogram and determined I needed angioplasty to unclog a blocked artery. While they were working on me, they tore my artery a bit and needed to put a stent in to repair it. It was just a small artery that was blocked and, fortunately, the damage to my heart was minor, so I was released a few days later with the warning that there was a significant risk of it clogging again.

My fiancé and I got married as planned on Maui three months later. It was there that I had my first panic attack. Can you blame me? I was worrying constantly about my heart. Doctors couldn't explain why I'd developed heart disease. Smoking and taking birth control pills together was the only thing that doctors said was a possible cause, but given my age, it was unlikely that these things alone caused my heart attack. One doctor even said, "Well, I guess you're just unlucky."

I'd made some changes to my lifestyle. I quit smoking—pretty easy to do when the doctor says that I'll be back in the hospital within three months if I keep it up. I was monitoring my eating better to reduce my cholesterol levels, and I was walking twice a day. So I didn't have any problems with my heart for a while, but now I was having panic attacks. For me, that was the worst part. I knew my heart was repaired, but I couldn't help worrying about every new ache and pain. The symptoms I was getting from panic attacks were so similar to those that I experienced during the heart attack that I spent many hours in the emergency room, scared that my heart was in trouble again. My panic attacks were unpredictable. I could have one even when I was doing something as monotonous as unloading the dishwasher.

I sought help from several doctors, who wanted me to take anxiety medication, but I resisted because I didn't want to be dependent on a mood-altering drug. I was referred to a six-week panic attack class. I remember the therapist describing panic symptoms. She said, "Many times when you panic the muscles in your chest tense up and cause pain. So when you feel that, you've got to know that it's not going to kill you, it's just your muscles. Well, except for you, Dawn. You've got to take that seriously." She also informed us that, "When you're short of breath, you're just hyperventilating yourself; it's not going to kill you. Except for you, Dawn." Obviously, that didn't apply to my situation either. The symptoms for a heart attack and a panic attack are so similar. So every time I had a panic attack, I'd freak out about my heart. I didn't know which was which.

I reluctantly decided that I was going to have to give the anxiety medications a try. I didn't want to be dependent on them, but I've found that they have given me some of my confidence back. I feel much better mentally but am now dealing with one of the most common side effects of anxiety/depression drugs—weight gain.

A year and seven months had passed since my heart attack. In December of 2002 I got some abnormal test results back. My doctor said it was a small area that was affected, and it could be a false positive. He said he wasn't worried about it and didn't further check my heart. Well, three months later, I was back in the hospital for another angioplasty and another stent. About a year later I was having shortness of breath. I was sent for a treadmill test that I didn't do well on. The doctor said that I was fine; I just needed to get in better shape. Again, he didn't further test my heart. Several months later I was back in the hospital for yet another procedure. The stent had clogged up almost completely. They placed two more stents in my artery to open it up. In addition, the doctor who worked on me accidentally tore a major artery, the left main coronary artery and had to stent it too in order to repair it. I now have five stents and am hoping that the third time is the charm.

My husband and I really want to start a family, but

the doctors are telling us that I shouldn't risk a pregnancy because it would be too hard on my heart. After all that we've been through, it was a heartbreaking thing to hear. We are hopeful of finding someone willing to be a surrogate mother for us. In the meantime, we are taking each day as it comes and meeting each new challenge as it arises.

I have now been symptom-free for over a year and a half, and I am hoping that this lasts for a while. I'm trying to keep my spirits up; I know I have been blessed several times over with another chance at life. Now, at thirty-three, I'm trying to use my experiences to make a positive difference. As a teacher, I show my students how to take care of their hearts. I talk to others and give them support as they go through their own battles with heart disease. I have become a spokesperson for the American Heart Association in the hope of inspiring other young women to understand and learn their risks of heart disease.

What I hope people learn from my story is that heart disease is indiscriminate when it comes to age, gender, or health. It is not just an old man's affliction. It can happen to anyone, at any time. Be aware of your body. Know the signs and symptoms. And don't ever assume that you're immune to heart disease. You're not.

Appendix

Straight from the Heart

*Resources for Women
with Heart Disease*

DIAGNOSTIC TEST

According to several doctors interviewed for this book, the ultrafast CT scan is probably the best diagnostic test for heart disease. If your health-insurance company does not want to pay for the test, you might consider paying for it yourself. Call 800–NEW–TEST.

HEART DISEASE–RELATED
ORGANIZATIONS AND WEB SITES

Events of the Heart

www.eventsoftheheart.org

Come and see the true stories in *Take It to Heart* adapted for the stage and performed by well-known celebrities. "Events" is a benefit to raise money for awareness, education, and research for women and heart disease. Traveling to major cities; check Web site for schedules.

WomenHeart: The National Coalition
for Women with Heart Disease

www.womenheart.org

Phone: 202–728–7199

The best advocacy organization with the coolest women who've had heart disease—your instant friends and future support network. Also a great Web site featuring the latest news, health brochures, and items to buy, such as the survival heart charm and red dress pin for heart disease. Women-Heart, in conjunction with the Mayo Clinic, also offers a training program for women to learn how to spread the word about heart disease in their local communities. Contact them for membership, brochures, and more information.

American Heart Association

www.americanheart.org

Phone: 888–MY–HEART

Funds medical research studies on heart disease. Web site offers comprehensive information about various heart conditions and treatments. Sponsors a public-awareness campaign for women about heart disease prevention, "Go Red for Women." Call to purchase the campaign's educational materials or download them from the Web.

National Heart, Lung, and Blood Institute (NHLBI)

www.nhlbi.nih.gov

Phone: 301–592–8573

Part of the National Institutes of Health. Sponsors "The Heart Truth" campaign, which features the Red Dress as the national symbol for women and heart disease. Call to order copies of campaign materials or view on-line. Publications include:

- *The Healthy Heart Handbook for Women*
- *The Heart Truth for Women: An Action Plan*
- *The Heart Truth for African-American Women: An Action Plan*
- *The Heart Truth for Latinas: An Action Plan*
- *When Delicious Meets Nutritious: Recipes for Heart Health*
- *Question to Ask Your Doctor/What's Your Risk?*

HeartCenterOnline

www.heartcenteronline.com

Click on the "Patients" icon to read information and the latest news about heart disease, risk factors, treatments, and the stories of other people with heart disease. You can sign up for free weekly E-mail newsletters devoted to heart disease and treatment, which are great updates. Also, they have a very active community bulletin board for chatting with other heart disease patients.

Heart Point

www.heartpoint.com

Click on "Gallery" to view a series of very cool animated articles about various heart conditions, treatments, and prevention methods. It also has heart-healthy recipes. A really fun site!

Mended Hearts

www.mendedhearts.org

Phone: 888–HEART–99

This national network of support groups for people recovering from heart bypass surgery and other procedures is affiliated with the American Heart Association. Visit their Web site or call for more information.

Heart Information Network

www.heartinfo.com

Offers comprehensive information on heart disease in the form of easy-to-read guides. Especially helpful are the sections marked "FAQs," which contain answers to top questions about heart disease, and "Health Encyclopedia," which explains medical jargon.

The Mayo Clinic

www.mayoclinic.com

Go to the Heart Disease Center under the "Diseases & Conditions" tab for fabulous up-to-date news, tools to test your risk, and an "Ask a Mayo Clinic doctor" section.

OTHER HEART DISEASE–RELATED ORGANIZATIONS TO CONTACT INCLUDE:

American College of Cardiology
American Society of Hypertension
American Stroke Association
Heart Failure Society of America
Pulmonary Hypertension Association
Adult Congenital Heart Association
Heart Rhythm Society
Preeclampsia Foundation

GENERAL MEDICAL INFORMATION AND WOMEN'S HEALTH–RELATED ORGANIZATIONS

Agency for Healthcare Research and Quality
www.ahrq.gov
Phone: 800–358–9295

The AHRQ publishes comprehensive clinical practice guidelines on heart disease (and other medical conditions) by panels of leading medical experts, which describe the latest knowledge and cutting-edge treatment guidelines for health-care professionals to follow. They are good reference guides, especially if you think you may not be getting the best medical care available. Less technical patient and family guides are also available. Download from the Web site or order by calling the toll-free number.

Society for Women's Health Research
www.womenshealthresearch.org

The nation's only nonprofit organization whose sole mission is to improve the health of women through research. It advocates increased funding for research on women's health issues; encourages the study of gender differences that may affect the prevention, diagnosis, and treatment of disease; and promotes the inclusion of women in medical research studies.

National Women's Health Information Center
www.4women.gov
The U.S. government's primary information site about women's health issues.

The National Women's Health Resource Center
www.healthywomen.org
A national clearinghouse of news, publications, and articles related to women's health issues.

MY FAVORITE HEART HEALERS

Joan Witkowski
Breath, energy, and conscious healing work
Phone: 212–620–0308

Fred Hahn
Owner, Serious Strength, Inc.
Phone: 212–579–9320

Dr. Gregory Costa
Chiropractor, homeopathy
Phone: 212–864–6127

Bruce Parker
Chiropractor
Phone: 310–456–7721

Oonaja Malagon
Yoga, quigong, energy healing
Phone: 845–657–6280

Micheline Berry
Yoga teacher—retreats and movement work
E-mail: micheline@zendancing.com

Liliya Chernova
Beauty therapist
Phone: 212–317–0925

John Steele
Master aromatherapist
Phone: 818–986–0594

Sally Kravich
Holistic nutritionist and iridologist
www.sallykravich.com
Phone: 212–946–1623 (New York City); 310–285–3528
(Los Angeles)

MY FAVORITE HEART PROFESSIONALS

Mark Budoff, M.D.
Phone: 310–222–4107
Associate professor of medicine, UCLA. Specializes in researching diagnostic tests for heart disease, such as the CT scan. An incredibly gifted cardiologist based in Los Angeles.

Jane Farhi, M.D.
Phone: 212–722–0854
Cardiologist, Lenox Hill Hospital, New York. She demonstrates unending patience and wisdom and is both internist and cardiologist.

Jesse Hanley, M.D.
www.jessehanleymd.com
E-mail: drhanley@jessehanleymd.com
Phone: 310–457–5806
Author of several books. Specializes in women's health, menopause, and integrating Eastern and Western medical approaches. She will get to the heart of what's going on and will explain it all beautifully. Private practice located in Malibu.

Alexandra Lanksy, M.D.

Assistant: Shannon Myers

E-mail: smyers@crf.org

Phone: 212–851–9322

Practicing cardiologist and associate professor at Columbia University Medical Center; director of the Cardiac Core Laboratories and the Women's Cardiovascular Health Initiative at the Cardiovascular Research Foundation. An amazing heart doctor.

Galina Mindlin, M.D., Ph.D.

www.brainmusictreatment.com

E-mail: info@brainmusictreatment.com

Phone: 212–888–2074

Conducts brain music therapy for depression, anxiety, stress, insomnia, and blood pressure issues. She will record your brain waves via EEG (noninvasive) and then create a CD that will both relax and energize you.

Beth Moran, A.R.N.P.

www.bethmoran.net

E-mail: bethnp@verizon.net

Phone: 941–351–3963

Nurse practitioner and holistic healer, as well as published author. She is sole proprietor of Integrated Wellness, a women's health-care practice in the Hamptons and Sarasota, Florida. She will take excellent care of your mind, body, and soul. She is full of life.

Erika Schwartz, M.D.
www.drerika.com
E-mail: info@drerika.com
Phone: 866–DR–ERICA
Author of several books, she makes frequent TV appearances. She is the guru of bioidentical hormones and menopause issues. She's also a great listener, problem solver, and women's advocate.

SHOP FOR THE CAUSE

The Sweetheart Bracelet
www.hearton.org
The symbol of *Heart On!* Designed by yours truly, author Pamela Serure herself. Give it to all the sweethearts in your life: mothers, wives, daughters, best friends, and yourself.

Also check for heart-friendly products and "Our Best of Heart List."

The Store at WomenHeart.org
www.womenheart.org/our_store.asp
The red dress pin, pendant, pashmina scarf, and tie, as well as books, cards, and posters related to heart disease.

BOOKS TO RECOVER BY

- *Essential Rumi,* by Coleman Barks. A Rumi a day keeps the blues away.
- *Letters to a Young Poet,* by Rainer Maria Rilke, translated by Stephen Mitchell. I reread this piece every year, especially letter #8.
- *Serve It Forth,* by M. F. K. Fisher. Fabulous for the literary gourmand.
- *Cries of the Spirit,* edited by Marilyn Sewell. The best compilation of poetry (my favorite is "Wild Geese," by Mary Oliver).
- *The Light Inside the Dark,* by John Tarrant Harper. Definitely a light inside the dark tunnel of recovery.
- *Heart: A Natural History of the Heart-Filled Life,* by Gail Goodwin. An interesting perspective.
- *Parabola: Myth, Tradition, and the Search for Meaning,* published by the Society for Study of Myth and Tradition. This quarterly publication offers spiritually based stories that always seem to offer exactly what I need to read at that moment.
- *Stories from the Heart: WomenHeart Patients Describe their Disease, Treatment, and Recovery,* compiled and arranged by Anastasia Roussos and Melissa Lausin. A collection of heart stories written

by the women themselves. They touch the heart
every time.

- *Twenty Love Poems and a Song of Despair,* by Pablo
Neruda. With a glass of red wine, this is a
perfect date.
- *Only Love Is Real: A Story of Soulmates Reuinted,* by
Brian Weiss, M.D. Dream and believe.
- *Start Where You Are: A Guide to Compassionate
Living,* by Pema Chodron. She always guides you
gently back to your self.
- *The Prophet,* by Khalil Gibran. A classic to comfort
the soul.
- *Loving What Is: Four Questions That Can Change
Your Life,* by Byron Katie, with Stephen Mitchell.
A new way to see who you are by what and who
you project on life.
- *A Heart as Wide as the World: Stories on the Path of
Lovingkindness,* by Sharon Salzberg. For inspiring
devoted contemplation.
- *Heart Sense for Women: Your Plan for Natural
Prevention and Treatment,* by Stephen T. Sinatra,
M.D.
- *Heartbreak and Heart Disease: A Mind/Body
Prescription for Healing the Heart,* by Stephen T.
Sinatra, M.D.

MUSIC TO RECOVER BY

- "Believe I Can Fly," Yolanda Adams, *The Experience*
- "A Change Is Gonna Come," Leela James, *A Change Is Gonna Come*
- "Feeling Good," Nina Simone, *Six Feet Under* (sound track)
- "Amazing Grace," Walela, *Walela*
- "Mercy Now," Mary Gauthier, *Mercy Now*
- "Love and Happiness," Al Green, *Greatest Hits*
- "Anniversary Song," Eva Cassidy, *Time After Time*
- "Anyone Who Had a Heart," Dusty Springfield, *The Ultimate Collection*
- "At Last," Chantal Chamberland, *Serendipity Street*
- "Avinu Malkeinu," Barbra Streisand, *Higher Ground*
- "Blue Moon Revisited (Song for Elvis)," Cowboy Junkies, *Best of Cowboy Junkies*
- "California Dreamin'," the Mamas and the Papas, *California Dreamin'*
- "Calling All Angels," Jane Siberry, with k.d. lang, *When I Was a Boy*
- "Me to the End of Love," Leonard Cohen, *Leonard Cohen Live in Concert*
- "Do You Want to Dance?," Bette Midler, *The Divine Miss M*

- "Don't Go Breaking My Heart," Elton John, *Greatest Hits 1970–2002*
- "Every Breath You Take," the Police, *Synchronicity*
- "Fly Me to the Moon," Dinah Washington, *Torch Songs* (disc 2)
- "Hecho a la Medida," Paulina Carraz, *Paulina Carraz*
- "Heaven Must Have Sent You," Bonnie Pointer, *The Best of the Pointer Sisters*
- "How High the Moon," Dianne Reeves, *I Remember*
- "I Believe/You'll Never Walk Alone," Barbra Streisand, *Higher Ground*
- "I Can't Make It Anymore," Richie Havens, *Mixed Bag*
- "I Will Survive," Chantay Savage, *Natural Woman* (volume 2, disc 1)
- "I've Fallen in Love with You," Joss Stone, *The Soul Sessions*
- "If I Could Turn Back the Hands of Time," R. Kelly, *R.* (disc 1)
- "If You Go Away," Shirley Bassey, *The Remix Album: Diamonds Are Forever*
- "In My Secret Life," Leonard Cohen, *Ten New Songs*
- "Into the Mystic," Van Morrison, *Moondance*

- "It's All Coming Back to Me Now," Celine Dion, *Falling into You*
- "It's Time," Linda Eder, *It's Time*
- "Just Like a Woman," Richie Havens, *Mixed Bag*
- "Lay Lady Lay," the Brothers and Sisters, *Dylan's Gospel*
- "Like a Lover," Dianne Reeves, *I Remember*
- "Love's Divine," Seal, *Grammy Nominees 2005*
- "Make Someone Happy," Jimmy Durante, *As Time Goes By*
- "My Heart Will Go On," Celine Dion, *Titanic* (sound track)
- "My Way (A Mi Manera)," Il Divo, *Il Divo*
- "One Fine Day," Natalie Merchant, *One Fine Day*
- "Prayer (For Kahlil Gibran)," Michael Hoppé and Martin Tillmann, *The Poet: Romances for Cello*
- "Samba Pa Ti," Santana, *Greatest Hits*
- "Somewhere Over the Rainbow," Patti Labelle, *Live!*
- "And I Love Her," the Beatles, *A Hard Day's Night*
- "The Best 4:10," Tina Turner, *Simply the Best*
- "The Blower's Daughter," Damien Rice, *O*
- "The First Cut Is the Deepest," Sheryl Crow, *Grammy Nominees 2005*
- "The Power of Love," Jennifer Rush, *The Power of Love*
- "The Way of Love," Cher, *Greatest Hits*

- "Timeless Motion," Daniel Kobialka, *Timeless Motion*
- "Total Eclipse of the Heart," Bonnie Tyler, *Faster Than the Speed of Night*
- "Thy Will Jaya Bagavan," Cloe Goodchild, *Devi*
- "Wild Is the Wind," David Bowie, *Golden Years*
- "Pavane for a Dead Princess," Deodato, *Deodato 2*
- "Gayatri Mantra," Deva Premal, *The Essence*
- "The Nearness of You / Misty," Dianne Reeves, *I Remember*
- "Night and Day," Frank Sinatra, *Sinatra Sings Cole Porter*
- "Hallelujah," Jeff Buckley, *Grace*
- "The Closest Thing to Crazy," Katie Melua, *Call Off the Search*
- "This Is True," Marisa Tomei, *A Gift of Love II*
- "Flight (For Robert Frost)," Michael Hoppé, *The Poet: Romances for Cello*
- "Autumn Leaves / When October Goes," Nancy LaMott, *Come Rain or Come Shine*
- "I Put A Spell on You," Nina Simone, *Don't Let Me Be Misunderstood*
- "Miracle (Radio Edit)," Olive, *Miracle*
- "Try a Little Tenderness," Paul Giamatti and Arnold McCuller, *Duets* (sound track)
- "Solos," Paulina Carraz, *Paulina Carraz*

- "Amado Mio," Pink Martini, *Sympathique*
- "Trouble," Ray LaMontagne, *Trouble*
- "Pavane," Regina Carter Paganini, *After a Dream*
- "Cinema Paradiso," Regina Carter Paganini, *After a Dream*
- "Unchained Melody," the Righteous Brothers, *The Best of the Righteous Brothers*
- "I Want to Know What Love Is," Wynonna Judd, *What the World Needs Now Is Love*
- "If It's Magic," Stevie Wonder, *Songs in The Key of Life* (disc 2)
- "Hallelujah," Angelou, *Sweet Dreams Tonight*
- "Adagio," Albinoni, *Greatest Hits of 1720*
- "Ave Maria," Chloe Goodchild, *Devi*
- "Goin' Out of My Head," Queen Latifah, *Living Out Loud*
- "I Am What I Am," Dido, *No Angel*
- "I Did It My Way," Elvis Presley, *Aloha from Hawaii*
- "I Put a Spell on You," Nina Simone, *Don't Let Me Be Misunderstood*
- "I'll Be Seeing You," Jane Monheit, *Come Dream with Me*
- "In My Heart," Moby, *18*
- "Mi Corazon," Gipsy Kings, *Tierra Gitana*
- "Namah Shivaya," Krishna Das, *Pilgrim Heart*
- "Unbreak My Heart," Toni Braxton, *Secrets*

- "One," U2, *The Family Man* (sound track)
- "I Will Always Love You," Whitney Houston, *The Bodyguard* (sound track)
- "What'll I Do," Chris Botti, *When I Fall in Love*
- "Suzanne," Judy Collins, *Forever: Anthology* (disc 1)

MY FAVORITE HEALING QUOTES

I have never met a person whose greatest need was anything other than real, unconditional love. You can find it in a simple act of kindness toward someone who needs help. There is no mistaking love. You feel it in your heart. It is the common fiber of life, the flame that heals our soul, energizes our spirit, and supplies passion to our lives. It is our connection to God and to each other.

—Elisabeth Kübler-Ross

We act as though comfort and luxury were the chief requirements of life, when all that we need to make us really happy is something to be enthusiastic about.

—Charles Kingsley

The greatest weakness of most humans is their hesitancy to tell others how much they love them while they're alive.

—AUTHOR UNKNOWN

God always answers in the deeps, never in the shallows of our soul.

—AUTHOR UNKNOWN

Everyone should carefully observe which way his heart draws him, and then choose that way with all his strength.

—HASIDIC SAYING

Who looks outside, dreams. Who looks inside, awakens.

—CARL JUNG

To understand the heart and mind of a person, look not at what he has already achieved, but at what he aspires to.

—KHALIL GIBRAN

You will find as you look back upon your life that the moments when you have truly lived are the moments when you have done things in the spirit of love.

—HENRY DRUMMOND

*I am the feminine qualities: fame, beauty, perfect
speech, memory, intelligence, loyalty, and forgiveness.*

—BHAGAVAD-GITA

*Everyone is so afraid of death, but the real sufis just
laugh: nothing tyrannizes their hearts. What strikes the
oyster shell does not damage the pearl.*

—RUMI

*All emotions are pure which gather you and lift you up;
that emotion is impure which seizes only one side of
your being and so distorts you.*

—RAINER MARIA RILKE

*For one human being to love another: that is perhaps
the most difficult of all our tasks; the ultimate, the last
test and proof, the work for which all other work is but
preparation.*

—RAINER MARIA RILKE

*I postpone death by living, by suffering, by error, by
risking, by giving, by losing.*

—ANAÏS NIN

*Look for a long time at what pleases you, and longer
still at what pains you.*

—COLLETTE

One is not born a woman, but becomes one.

—SIMONE DE BEAUVOIR

It isn't until you come to a spiritual understanding of who you are—not necessarily a religious feeling, but deep down, the spirit within—that you can begin to take control.

—OPRAH WINFREY

If you do not bring forth what is within you, what is within you will destroy you.

—THE GOSPEL OF ST. THOMAS

ACKNOWLEDGMENTS

To my beloved Cheyenne, who came into my heart and never let it go, who supplies endless moments of nourishment, guidance, and care for my soul. I thank you for standing in the fire without shrinking back and for sharing your courage with me. To the amazing Dr. Jesse Hanley, who through her intuition and medical acumen figured out that my heart needed to be fixed. For her countless hours of generosity and gentle care, thank you for the sunny days in my time of gloom. To Donna Karan for being my sister in the time when I needed one most. To Sage, somewhere in heaven and always in my heart.

To Geneen for her endless cups of tea and bowls of chicken soup, and for taking charge with all her heart and being so lovely in a time of terror. To K.T., who always brought hope, joy, and a sense that my adventures weren't over yet. To Mo, who bought me a computer and knew I had to write this story. To Virginia, my sweet shaman of dreams, for teaching me the wisdom of my suffering and being my midwife. To Marlette and Raymond for being so close and such loving family. To my brother, Teddy, for being so my brother. To Rabbi Judith, who through her prayers and teaching brought me to believe in the grace of it all. Thank you also to all my new friends in L.A., who helped me navigate the hills, valleys, wind, and rain: Denise, Tim, Victoria, Chantal, Linda, Lucy, Cedric, Michael, Joy, Paula, and Patricia, Sue, Joann, Gil, Shirley, Susan, and Sybil. To all the body workers who nourished me, stretched me, massaged me, and put me back together: Micheline, Bruce, Selso, Edie, and the New York masters Oonaja and Gregory.

To Laura Yorke, my agent, with her laser-sharp wit and acumen in helping me make sense out of my story. I so appreciate her ability to get things done in a New York minute. To Carol Mann, who also represented this book, even when the tides were turning away from it. To MeiMei Fox, the editor who made order out of my life's chaos, blending the ingredients into the most perfect soup. I cherish your heart and the way you put it into this book. To my publisher, Amy Hertz, who had the compassion and the vision to see my individual story and know it was for Everywoman, and for easing my suffering by allowing this story to be written. My heart will always be grateful to you for bringing to light everything about heart disease that was hidden in the dark.

To all the doctors who prodded, poked, and pulled me through: Dr. John Robinson for your precision, Dr. William Coke Harrell for meditating with me during my recovery, Dr. Richard Taw for your expediency, Carolyn Conger for your wisdom and grace, Brugh Joy for never leaving anything to chance, and Dr. Sharonne Hayes for making women's hearts the priority and demanding the best for us. To Dr. Jane Farhi, who ushered me to safety when I needed another procedure, thank you for letting me come in whenever I needed reassurance. To Dr. Erika Schwartz, who connects the dots from my head to my heart. And to my group from WomenHeart, the ladies who lunch with all their heart: Sylvia, Debby, Maria, Connie, Maxine, and Belinda. Also to Nancy Loving for shepherding WomenHeart and corralling all the women who needed support together. You are a force and an inspiration.

To those friends who have heard my story so many times and still make me feel brand-new. To friends and family members who have lent me a hand and a heart to lean on, money to assist my healing, inspiration to rest on, and cushions for all my blows. To my custodians of laughter and emergency rooms, Heide and Howard. To Maxi for providing a safe, creative environment when I needed it most. To Joe, Kenny, and Stan Cayre, the most generous of brothers; to Jack B., Harry A., and Sol W. for being mensches; to

Miriam and her healing teas; to Sharamie, Nancy B., Rosie; and finally to Josh, Lenore, and Zach and Pavi for voting me in. And to my hero, Hoot, who saved me more than a few times. To Helene Lerner, who always champions women's causes. To Arielle and Debby for their total heart support. To all the women of NAFE and their incredible network of strength and support. To Betty Spense for shepherding the herd. To all the nurses who patiently and lovingly cared for me during all those days of trauma. And to Jimmy, who is the best father to Habebe.

To all the women who have contributed your stories to this book, I wish you all the courage to keep on going. And finally to all those women whom I have yet to meet who will soon come forward with their heart stories.